Fundamentals of Decentralized
Clinical Trials

Anna H. Yang
Isaac R. Rodriguez-Chavez
Editors

Fundamentals of Decentralized Clinical Trials

Strategy and Execution

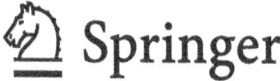

Editors
Anna H. Yang, PharmD
Principal Clinical Innovation and
Technology Leader
Genentech, A Member of the
Roche Group (United States)
South San Francisco, CA, USA

Isaac R. Rodriguez-Chavez, PhD
CEO & Principal Independent
Consultant, Scientific, Clinical
Regulatory Affairs and Digital
Health Technologies
4Biosolutions Consulting
Rockville, MD, USA

ISBN 978-3-031-62879-5   ISBN 978-3-031-62877-1   (eBook)
https://doi.org/10.1007/978-3-031-62877-1

© The Editor(s) (if applicable) and The Author(s), under exclusive license to Springer Nature Switzerland AG 2024, corrected publication 2024
This work is subject to copyright. All rights are solely and exclusively licensed by the Publisher, whether the whole or part of the material is concerned, specifically the rights of translation, reprinting, reuse of illustrations, recitation, broadcasting, reproduction on microfilms or in any other physical way, and transmission or information storage and retrieval, electronic adaptation, computer software, or by similar or dissimilar methodology now known or hereafter developed.
The use of general descriptive names, registered names, trademarks, service marks, etc. in this publication does not imply, even in the absence of a specific statement, that such names are exempt from the relevant protective laws and regulations and therefore free for general use.
The publisher, the authors and the editors are safe to assume that the advice and information in this book are believed to be true and accurate at the date of publication. Neither the publisher nor the authors or the editors give a warranty, expressed or implied, with respect to the material contained herein or for any errors or omissions that may have been made. The publisher remains neutral with regard to jurisdictional claims in published maps and institutional affiliations.

This Springer imprint is published by the registered company Springer Nature Switzerland AG
The registered company address is: Gewerbestrasse 11, 6330 Cham, Switzerland

If disposing of this product, please recycle the paper.

Foreword

Decentralized clinical trials predated the COVID-19 pandemic, but the urgency to sustain research during the pandemic was an overwhelming catalyst for adoption. While adoption curves of change and innovation in clinical research are typically measured in years, decentralized research methods have aggressively moved toward meaningful adoption in a matter of months. Now comes the hard work of sustaining, scaling, and generating the evidence of impact essential to maintain momentum. With such a rapid state of change in operational strategies, regulatory intelligence and experience feedback from site staff and participants alike, it may be hard to imagine how to codify learnings in a book. It is ambitious to attempt to capture this state of operations, technology, and intelligence for publication while appreciating how much learning is still taking place. And yet, a book is exactly what is needed to maintain learning and continue to grow the research community as ready and empowered to embrace decentralized research and improve access and participation for all.

Decentralized Trials and Research Alliance Craig Lipset
San Diego, CA, USA

Former Head, Clinical Innovation, Pfizer
New York City, NY, USA

Preface

Welcome to the world of decentralized clinical trials (DCTs), where innovation meets necessity, and traditional paradigms in clinical research are being reshaped. In the ever-evolving landscape of healthcare, the need for more flexible and patient-centric approaches to clinical trials has become increasingly apparent. This short handbook, *Fundamentals of Decentralized Clinical Trials: Strategy and Execution*, hopes to serve as your comprehensive guide to understanding the fundamental principles, strategies, and execution of DCT methods.

In Chap. 1: Introduction, we delve into the catalysts driving the adoption of DCT approaches, particularly amidst the backdrop of the COVID-19 pandemic. We explore the significant financial, structural, and strategic investments made in the industry, shedding light on pivotal DCTs that have paved the way for transformative learnings.

In Chap. 2: Technology Landscape and Requirements, we traverse through the intricate web of digital transformation within clinical trials. For those unfamiliar with the terrain of health data interoperability and technological innovations, this chapter serves as a beacon of insight. By unraveling the complexities of the technology landscape, our aim is to arm future clinical trials researchers with the confidence to navigate through unfamiliar terminologies and embrace the digital evolution shaping the field.

Navigating the regulatory landscape is paramount in ensuring the success and compliance of DCTs. Chapter 3 provides an in-depth analysis of the regulatory framework, with a particular focus on the draft FDA guidance released in May 2023. Authored by leading experts in the field, this chapter offers invaluable insights into navigating the regulatory intricacies inherent in DCT execution.

As we delve deeper into the methodology of trial design and implementation in Chap. 4, we explore the multifaceted implications of DCT approaches on trial teams. From redefining trial methodologies to garnering early feedback from Ethics Committees and Investigational Review Boards, this chapter elucidates the transformative impact of decentralized methodologies on traditional trial paradigms.

Finally, in Chap. 5: Goals and Metrics of Success, we contemplate the metrics by which the success of DCT approaches is measured. As an early exploration into this burgeoning field, this chapter provides a snapshot of the industry's evolving perspectives on measuring key performance indicators, with the understanding that further insights will continue to emerge.

In closing, this handbook serves as both a primer for embracing the future of clinical research. Whether you are a seasoned industry professional or a budding researcher, "Fundamentals of Decentralized Clinical Trials: Strategy and Execution" equips you with the knowledge and insights needed to navigate the dynamic landscape of DCTs with confidence and foresight.

Best regards,

South San Francisco, CA, USA   Anna H. Yang

The original version of the book has been revised. A correction to this book can be found at https://doi.org/10.1007/978-3-031-62877-1_6

Introduction by Anna H. Yang

Thank you to all the industry researchers before me who have been the ones to be bold, share their ideas, and publish their data. The field of decentralized clinical trials (DCTs) has changed enormously since I started working on it in 2019. This short handbook is for the eager learners like me, 4 years ago, who seek to understand and get up to speed on what DCTs mean and how to work in this space. As you can imagine, it is difficult to collate the relevant evidence around a rapidly evolving topic. Despite the first DCT being executed in 2001, the evolution and widespread industry adoption didn't really start until the COVID-19 pandemic. Therefore, as of 2023, I believe we are still in the very early stages of understanding and implementing technology solutions and innovative services in our trials. There are also different indicators—lagging data versus current data versus leading data—and for the sake of including the right information our authors have decided to include the lagging data, primarily peer-reviewed, published data. This is just one version of the story. We will continue to iterate on the content. I believe we have the right thought leaders today to review the information.

Thank you for your curiosity. I hope you find this information helpful and invite you to embark on the journey with us. May your ideas help us reshape the content of this book for future versions.

South San Francisco, CA, USA Anna H. Yang

Introduction
by Isaac R. Rodriguez-Chavez

I am delighted to introduce this book on DCTs, offering a thorough exploration of their potential to revolutionize clinical research through innovative technology. DCTs, as discussed in Chap. 1, address barriers to traditional trial participation, promoting accessibility, diversity, equity, and participant engagement. Chapter 2 examines how the COVID-19 pandemic and evolving regulations accelerated the adoption of DCTs, building on their application since the early 2000s. Chapters 3 and 4 highlight remaining operational complexities and the importance of careful trial design to ensure scientific rigor, operational feasibility, and compliance with regulations, ethics, data privacy, and participant safety. The book emphasizes the significance of the FDA's draft guidance on DCTs, detailing investigator responsibilities, local health providers' use, and essential sponsor considerations. Chapter 5 stresses the need for clear metrics to evaluate DCT adoption's impact on recruitment, retention, diversity, safety, and cost efficiencies. These measures are pivotal in objectively assessing the value and sustainability of decentralized models. Chapters 1 and 5 underscore the importance of meeting participants' geographic and emotional needs, unlocking broader trial populations while maintaining safety and data integrity. Embracing pragmatic DCT adoption, either alongside traditional methods or hybrid models, is crucial, placing the participant experience at the forefront while maintaining safety and clinical data quality and integrity. This guide tracks DCT advancements and encourages readers to contribute to evidence-based integration, meeting participant expectations for convenience and fostering faster, more inclusive trials. Ultimately, this book aims to support the transformation of modern clinical research, developing medical products more efficiently for those in need.

Rockville, MD, USA   Isaac R. Rodriguez-Chavez

Acknowledgments

Thank you, first and foremost, to all patients for their immense courage and selflessness to advance human health.

Thank you to Genentech/Roche, for supporting me in this side project for the field.

Thank you, colleagues, for making this book a success:

Rasika Kalamegham, Sharad Nair, Eric Lin, Paul Wilds, Kimberly Barnholt, Seema Asthana, Beverly Assman, Nikheel Kolatar, Janet Moga, Carmen Leung, James Wilson, Arjun Tyagi, Courtney Tegler, Rena Liu-Critchley, Amy Vassel, Patricia Mader

Barnabé Lecouteux, Tammy Jackson, Amy Apostoleris, Will Lee, Nan Croy, Fabien Didier, Stuart Redding, Brian Bush, Sujit Nair, Justin Chickles, Kristina Reeder, John Manns, Claudine Paccio, Paige Altrogge

Kenneth Getz, Micky Tripathi, Stephen Konya, Caroline Redeker

To my family and friends, thank you:

Richard Laux, my loving partner, for your unwavering encouragement and reminders to embrace joy and celebration.

My parents Yisong Yang and Sheng Wang, my twin sister Julia, and my older brother Peter for their wisdom and for consistently showing me the essence of perseverance and dedication.

Channy Chhi-Laux, Kent Laux, and Natasha Laux, for their love and support throughout our journey.

- My previous boss and dear friend, Marianne Chacon-Araya, for believing in me as a Fellow and giving me free reign to experiment throughout my creative processes.
- My best friends, Brenda, Carolyn, Irene, and Connie, for being my squad and for cheering me on.
- The "BroHub," Chris, Rob, Ro, James, Sapna, PK, and Steph, for their insights and radical candor.

Contents

1 **Introduction and Overview of Decentralized Clinical Trials** 1
Anna H. Yang, Marianne Chacon-Araya, and Jane Myles
Evolving Need for Decentralized Clinical Trials Prior to the COVID-19 Pandemic.................. 2
Catalysts During the COVID-19 Pandemic That Accelerated Decentralized Clinical Trial Adoption...................................... 3
Financial, Structural and Strategic Investments Made in the Industry........................... 6
Defining Decentralized Clinical Trials and Key Digital Health Technologies............... 7
Industry Trends, Notable Decentralized Clinical Trials, Their Key Successes and Lessons Learned for the Industry 9
Bibliography 13

2 **Technology Landscape and Requirements** 17
Anna H. Yang and Isaac R. Rodriguez-Chavez
Data Flow Between Systems in a Clinical Trial 18
  Introduction to Findable, Accessible, Interoperable and Reusable Data Principles........ 18
Health Data Interoperability and US-Based Efforts to Harmonize Adoption................... 21

xv

	Technology Implementation Considerations	25
	Technology Components	26
	List Predictions and Future Trends for Emerging Cross-Industry Trends..........................	29
	Bibliography	32
3	**Regulatory Landscape**	35
	Isaac R. Rodriguez-Chavez and Anna H. Yang	
	Regulatory Stage Pre COVID-19 Pandemic..........	35
	Regulatory Adjustments During the COVID-19 Pandemic......................................	38
	Release of the FDA DCT Draft Guidance and Beyond...................................	41
	Reaffirming the Definition and Value of DCT	41
	DCT Design	42
	Remote Visits: Telehealth and Non-trial Personnel....................................	43
	Responsibilities of the Investigator...............	44
	Considerations for Investigational Product.........	44
	Looking Beyond	45
	Bibliography	47
4	**Methodology and Protocol Development**	49
	Anna H. Yang and Isaac R. Rodriguez-Chavez	
	Introduction to the Clinical Trial Team..............	50
	Clinical Research Team	50
	Impact of Decentralized Elements to the Trial Team....................................	52
	How Might a DCT Affect the Team?	52
	How to Write a Flexible Protocol for Decentralized Elements	53
	Trial Objectives and Trial Endpoints	54
	Trial Design...............................	55
	Inclusion and Exclusion Criteria.................	56
	Data Sources	56

Preparations Considerations for Ethics
Committees and Investigational Review Boards....... 57
   Multi-Regional Clinical Trials and Medable
   Task Force for IRB/EC Considerations
   for DCT Review 58
   Looking Ahead 60
Bibliography 62

5 Goals and Metrics of Success..................... 63
Isaac R. Rodriguez-Chavez, Anna H. Yang,
Jane Myles, and Shelly Barnes
Background and Commentary 64
Early Metrics of Success......................... 65
   Metric 1. Likelihood to Engage in a DCT 66
   Metric 2. Participant Dropout Percentage Due
   to Participant Decision 67
   Metric 3. Number of Adverse Events Reported
   Per Number of Randomized Participants 68
   Metric 4. Speed Through Enrollment Rate......... 68
   Metric 5. Diversity and Inclusion 69
   Metric 6. Cost 70
   Metric 7. Participant Load Per Site............... 71
   Metric 8. Database Lock Timelines 71
   Metric 9. Compliance 71
   Metric 10. Inclusion of Participants
   in a Clinical Trial Due to DCT Facility 72
Applying These Metrics to Trial Design............. 72
   Closing 73
Bibliography 75

**Correction to: Fundamentals of Decentralized
Clinical Trials** C1

Notes.. 77

Index.. 79

Introduction and Overview of Decentralized Clinical Trials

Anna H. Yang, Marianne Chacon-Araya, and Jane Myles

Objectives
By the end of this chapter, you will be able to:

1. Describe the evolving need for decentralized clinical trial (DCT) approaches prior to the COVID-19 pandemic.
2. Summarize the catalysts during the COVID-19 pandemic that accelerated adoption of DCT approaches.
3. Cite financial, structural, and strategic investments made from the pharmaceutical industry, contract research organizations, technology companies, and startups.
4. Define DCTs and key digital health terminologies.
5. Highlight trends, notable DCTs, and describe key successes and learnings for the industry.

A. H. Yang (✉)
Genentech, A Member of the Roche Group,
South San Francisco, CA, USA

M. Chacon-Araya
Pardes Biosciences, Carlsbad, CA, USA

J. Myles
Decentralized Trials and Research Alliance, San Diego, CA, USA
e-mail: jane.myles@dtra.org

© The Author(s), under exclusive license to Springer Nature Switzerland AG 2024
A. H. Yang, I. R. Rodriguez-Chavez (eds.), *Fundamentals of Decentralized Clinical Trials*,
https://doi.org/10.1007/978-3-031-62877-1_1

Evolving Need for Decentralized Clinical Trials Prior to the COVID-19 Pandemic

It is repeatedly estimated that fewer than 5% of all adult participants enroll in clinical trials across all disease areas [1, 2]. Reasons for lack of trial participation include geographic accessibility; financial, and cultural barriers; logistical concerns; clinical criteria; and a lack of resources for participants and clinicians to support enrollment and retention [3]. The 2021 Center for Information and Study on Clinical Research Participation (CISCRP) Participant Insights and Perceptions Survey highlights that knowing the trial's potential risks, benefits, purpose, and information on the trial drug are crucial for participants when deciding to participate in trials [4]. Certain subgroup populations identify specific barriers in this report; middle-aged respondents ages 45–64 place greater importance on flexible visit scheduling and number of trial visits than any other age subgroup. Black respondents are more likely to place greater importance on having both diverse staff and diverse participants than any other racial subgroup.

When nonmodifiable structural and clinical barriers are removed, around half of all participants who are offered to participate in a clinical trial enroll. A systematic review and meta-analysis of 35 oncology trials from 2000 through 2020 revealed that when given the opportunity to participate in a clinical trial, 55% of participants agreed to enroll. The main reasons for non-enrollment were the desire to control treatment choice and lack of interest. The authors concluded that interventions to improve participation should focus on modifiable factors: Accessibility and broadening eligibility criteria [5]. Otherwise, these barriers disproportionately affect certain groups: Older adults, medically underserved racial and ethnic groups, those of lower socioeconomic status (SES), participants with comorbidities, and rurally based residents [6]. Slow clinical trial recruitment is significantly costly and extends trial timelines. It is the number one reason for clinical trial premature termination [2, 5, 7]. Therefore, accessibility to trial participants and clinical trial enrollment speed have been highlighted as key drivers for faster scientific decision making to drive new treatments and innovative approaches in the clinical trial industry.

Global regulators are sending clear signals about their expectation to include the participant perspective in the design of clinical trials, and the need to include participants reflective of the real-world population in trials. These expectations set the foundation for a shift in traditional clinical trial design and execution approaches. In 2018, the United States Food and Drug Administration (FDA) released the "Participant-Focused Drug Development" final guidance, which provides a stepwise approach on how to submit participant experience data for drug regulatory decision-making [8]. In 2020, after decades of encouraging diversity enrollment practices, the FDA published the final guidance for "Enhancing Diversity of Clinical Trial Populations" to increase enrollment in underrepresented populations [9]. Together, these guidance documents and shifts in policy are driving a need to change trials and how they are conducted.

Catalysts During the COVID-19 Pandemic That Accelerated Decentralized Clinical Trial Adoption

The entire approach to healthcare delivery and clinical trials shifted when the coronavirus disease pandemic shook the world in late 2019. Patients and healthcare providers needed to self-isolate, non-critical in-person visits stopped, and patients with life-threatening illnesses experienced severe disruption in care. Participants' access to trial sites was reduced by 80% as health-system resources became consumed by coronavirus disease (COVID-19)-related care and travel became limited by physical distancing. The number of monthly trial-starts declined 50% at the beginning of the pandemic and low numbers persisted for the next 12 months. Many health systems and healthcare providers, including the Centers for Medicaid and Medicare Services (CMS) supported reimbursement for telehealth during this time. In the United States, all 50 states including Washington, D.C. passed licensure waivers that allowed participants to participate in telehealth visits with out-of-state clinicians. This benefitted participants in rural areas, according to an analysis conducted between 2017 and 2020 evaluating Medicare Beneficiaries [10]. Clinical care teams attempted to adopt remote participant monitoring for participants in the home setting recovering from COVID-19, or tracked participants recently discharged from an acute care setting. Flexibility in clinical care was not only possible but required, and the maturity of technology and remote services supported this model.

Around 1000 organizations reported trial disruption due to the pandemic and trialists reported an 80% decrease in new participants entering trials per site in April 2020 compared with April 2019 [11]. To preserve participant safety and trial integrity, the pharmaceutical industry found ways to accelerate trial innovations through decentralized clinical trial (DCT) approaches. FDA supported these flexible methods by publishing guidance documents in 2020, such as the "Conduct of Clinical Trials of Medical Products During the COVID-19 Public Health Emergency", "Statistical Considerations for Clinical Trials During COVID-19", and "Assessing COVID-19-Related Symptoms in Outpatient Adult and Adolescent Subjects in Clinical Trials of Drugs and Biological Products for COVID-19 Prevention or Treatment". Investigators that quickly adopted DCT approaches cited that the most-used DCT elements were digital participant engagement, trial virtualization, and site support. In order of importance, the specific methods are telehealth consultation, remote participant monitoring, remote trial initiation visits or investigator meetings, online participant recruitment, eConsent, and tools for site staff augmentation.

In May 2023, the FDA defined a DCT as a clinical trial where some (hybrid DCTs) or all (full DCTs) of the trial-related activities occur at locations other than traditional clinical trial sites that are headed by a qualified Investigator [12]. This definition aligns closely with the methods that the pharmaceutical industry has implemented to enable trial continuity. DCT approaches are not limited to technology and serve to enable flexibility and options for participants to participate in clinical research.

Even before COVID-19, the pharmaceutical industry emphasized the importance of reaching broad populations and "meeting participants where they are." For example, research suggests that geographic location may impact health outcomes. Rural residents are less likely to participate in clinical trial and experience more clinical and logistical barriers to medical care. In a trial of 7080 participants diagnosed with common cancers (breast, prostate, lung, colorectal), 1299 (18.5%) are from rural areas. Rural participants are more likely to have more than one comorbid condition (45.4% vs 39.5%), be more concerned with how to pay for their care (40.6% versus 32.4%), and travel farther for care (median 50.0 miles vs 12 miles) [5]. In colon cancer participants, increased travel burden is associated with decreased rates of receiving adjuvant chemotherapy. In a trial cohort of 34,694 stage III colon cancer trial participants, the odds ratio (OR) or likelihood of receiving adjuvant chemotherapy is 0.87 [0.78–0.96; $p = 0.009$], compared with 0.36 [0.28–0.45; $p < 0.001$] for participants who traveled 50 to 249 miles or beyond 250 miles to a treatment center [13]. DCT approaches can help remove these geographic barriers, address gaps that uniquely affect these populations, and reach a larger number and potentially more diverse pool of trial participants.

Pharmaceutical companies may use diverse DCT approaches to expedite participant recruitment, enhance retention rates, and boost participant adherence, potentially expediting trial completion. As consumers increasingly embrace digital technologies for everyday tasks like home deliveries, the expectation for similar convenience extends to their healthcare experiences as participants. DCTs, once considered innovative and cutting-edge, are now not just luxury options in clinical research but a crucial necessity and strategic approaches to flexible trial design and conduct for advancing medical product development with optimized efficiencies.

Financial, Structural and Strategic Investments Made in the Industry

During COVID-19 and the post-pandemic phase, many health technology vendors built platforms to support full and hybrid DCTs. These vendors offer end-to-end technology stack or service models that can be customized depending on the DCT need and be configured within a few months. This singular platform approach can offer advantages to sites, participants, and sponsors by decreasing the complexity associated with using multiple point solutions across several vendors. (e.g. eConsent, mobile nursing and eCOA each contracted with different service providers) to differentiate themselves in an ever-competitive market, some vendors have established strategic partnerships with clinical trial and data management platforms, contract research organizations (CROs), electronic health records (EHR) or health systems, data privacy/connectivity companies, consumer technology companies, and retail pharmacies.

- Clinical trial and data management partnerships streamline DCT operations and efficiency in data collection and management. Examples include: Medable and Parexel, Science37 and Clinical Research IO, Thread and Medidata.
- CRO partnerships enhance trial design and execution, particularly accelerating participant enrollment. Examples include: Deep Lens and IQVIA, Science37 and ICON, Evidation Health and PPD, Medable and Syneos.
- EHR partnerships integrate real-world data collection and extensive data collection abilities. Examples include: Evidation Health and Cerner, Thread and Oracle.
- Data connectivity partnerships enable secure and streamlined data sharing. Examples include: Medable and Datavant.
- Consumer technology partnerships would accelerate trial enrollment due to access to a large customer base. An example is Thread and Amazon Web Services.
- Retail pharmacy partnerships would accelerate participant recruitment and enable flexible remote visits. The only partner-

ship was Medable and CVS Clinical Trial Services, which unfortunately did not continue because CVS shut down their clinical trial services 2 years following launch.

These and other partnerships aim to increase trial efficacy and eliminate risks and delays while improving the experience for participants and site practitioners.

Defining Decentralized Clinical Trials and Key Digital Health Technologies

Clinical research can be divided into two broad categories: Non-interventional (e.g., observational studies, natural cohort studies, and retrospective or prospective cohort studies) and interventional clinical research (e.g., phase I–III clinical trials testing the safety and efficacy of an experimental medical product). As an example of non-interventional clinical research, an observational study is a type of clinical study in which individuals are observed or certain outcomes are measured. No attempt is made to affect the outcome (e.g., no treatment is given). In observational studies, investigators do not try to affect the outcome. They simply observe groups of people to determine associations between exposures and outcomes. Often, observational studies are the only feasible way to examine associations in humans between exposures and outcomes. Observational studies can also be called data collection studies or registry studies [14]. In contrast, in interventional clinical research, the investigator intervenes to prevent or treat a disease [15]. The DCT principles were originally developed for interventional clinical research, but they may be applied to non-interventional clinical research. Decentralized elements include electronic consent, telehealth, digital health tools, direct-to-participant shipment of investigational medical products (IMPs), home health care, and use of local healthcare providers (HCPs) and/or facilities [12, 16]. Public-private partnerships such as the Clinical Trials Transformation Initiative (CTTI) in the US and business consortiums such a Trials@Home in Europe have defined

DCTs to be operational and technology strategies to increase trial accessibility for participants in which some (hybrid DCTs) or all (full DCTs) assessments are conducted at locations other than the investigator site [17, 18]. DCTs also take advantage of flexible remote assessments, wherein the participant's care can be managed locally by their primary treating physician with virtual oversight by a remote primary investigator.

As described earlier, the US FDA definition of a DCT is a trial in which some (hybrid DCT) or all (full DCT) trial-related activities occur at locations other than traditional sites. This enables greater convenience to participants and may reduce burden to caregivers. Prior to the release of this official definition, DCTs were already similarly defined by a few early pre-competitive industry consortiums, including Clinical Trials Transformation Initiative (CTTI), Transcelerate, Decentralized Trials and Research Alliance (DTRA), Biotechnology Innovation Organization (BIO), Pharmaceutical Research and Manufacturers of America (PhRMA), commercial Institutional Review Boards (IRBs), and contract research organizations (CROs).

DCTs may leverage digital health technologies (DHTs). Digital health is defined as the application of digital technologies that help deliver and/or help provide access to healthcare products and services. Benefits of digital health extend beyond DCTs, such as the potential to accurately predict, diagnose, or prevent disease through the application of artificial intelligence (AI), machine learning (ML), and advanced analytics of large learning models. DCTs leverage digital health tools, such as telehealth, mobile health, health information technology, and wearables or devices (known as DHTs). Telehealth is defined as the use of telecommunications such as audiovisual conferencing (video calls) or audio conferencing (phone call) to provide remote care to participants in clinical trials without the need for an in-person office visit with the Investigator, Sub-Investigator, or appropriate and qualified trial personnel. Mobile health is defined by the Global Observatory of eHealth of the World Health Organization as "medical and public health practice supported by mobile devices, such as mobile phones, participant monitoring devices, personal digital assistants, and other wireless devices". Mobile health is a broad term that seems to also encompass DHTs (e.g., digital wearables, devices, and sensors). Health information technology is related to the storage, transfer, exchange, and process of health information in an electronic environment, which spans routine and clinical trial care. As an example, DHTs are equipment that may track biometric data, which includes but are not limited to heart rate, respiratory rate, sleep, activity, oxygen saturation, blood pressure, temperature, electrocardiogram (ECG), and any summarized applications of these scores. These technologies can contribute to tracking and measuring a participant's overall health and wellness (e.g., physical fitness trackers and watches) as well as assist with clinical decision making (e.g., blood pressure and ECG devices).

Industry Trends, Notable Decentralized Clinical Trials, Their Key Successes and Lessons Learned for the Industry

In 2007, the FDA and Duke University collaborated to form CTTI to modernize the way in which clinical trials were conducted [19]. In 2018, as part of the Mobile Clinical Trials (MCT) Program, CTTI released a recommendation for designing and conducting DCTs. This document distills actual and perceived challenges of legal, practical, and regulatory topics. It is widely recognized as the first high-level resource for Sponsors for comprehensive considerations in writing a protocol, how and who to engage with from a stakeholder perspective, cautionary watchouts for telehealth and clinical oversight across state borders, and recommendations for organizing chain of custody for IMP, to name a few. The document did not provide a roadmap for Sponsors on how to build towards a fully DCT nor metrics of success for what defines a successfully designed and executed DCT. The document provided a glimpse into the different options for hybrid DCTs—noting that a DCT does not have to be an "all-or-nothing" approach.

In 2001, Eli Lilly conducted the first randomized, placebo-controlled DCT that utilized the internet for the informed consent, randomization, and drug dispensing process. Eighty-three participants were enrolled and randomly assigned either tadalafil 20 mg or placebo for 4 weeks for the treatment of erectile dysfunction. The efficacy data resembled traditional tadalafil clinical trial data. The incidence of adverse events, however, was lower than anticipated. In a post-trial survey, 77% of participants who had traditional trial experience indicated that the DCT (coined "interactive clinical trial" back then) was better than a traditional trial [20].

In 2011, Pfizer initiated the REMOTE trial, in order to evaluate the safety and efficacy of tolterodine tartrate extended release (ER) 4 mg in participants with overactive bladder [21]. The trial's objective was to determine if the results from 600 participants could replicate the results of previously completed traditional phase IV trials of tolterodine tartrate ER. If the REMOTE trial succeeded, Pfizer would be able to prove that participants could engage in clinical trials without the need to visit physical sites. The REMOTE trial recruited participants from the web, screened participants using web-based questionnaires, obtained laboratory assessments in the community, and entered a run-in phase during e-diaries. Informed consent was obtained via the web and the medication was shipped directly to the participant's homes. Of the originally planned 600 participants, 5157 registered on the website, 456 passed screening, 237 passed medical screening, 118 entered the placebo run-in, and only 18 participants passed the e-diary assessments and were randomized to treatment [21].

The REMOTE trial's efforts were commended by Janet Woodcock, M.D., director of the Center for Drug Evaluation and Research at FDA at the time: "We commend Pfizer's progress on the REMOTE pilot and encourage all manufacturers considering other novel ideas in advancing clinical trials to have prospective discussions with the Agency regarding trial design and oversight". Despite low enrollment, the authors concluded that tolterodine tartrate ER showed similar efficacy and safety results compared to that of conventional trials, recommending a tweak of simplifying multi-step screening and testing [22].

The 2021 CISCRP Participant Perceptions and Insights Study around participant engagement identified that the increased use of technology and other convenience-enhancing initiatives—smart phone apps, text messaging, and video conferencing with trial doctors—were cited as most helpful. Additionally, a survey in

1183 participants conducted by the American Cancer Society from July 6, 2021 through September 8, 2021 showed that 60–85% of participants were more likely to enroll in a clinical trial if the trial used remote technology and other tools to decrease the need to travel to a site [23]. The survey also indicated that older participants (>55 years) and participants living in households of lower income (<$70,000) were more likely to benefit from remote participation, citing logistics and commute distance as major barriers to participation.

COVID-19 rapidly accelerated DCT adoption due to increased attention and evolving needs from participants, trial sites, and Sponsors [24]. Several sponsor companies converted their clinical trials during COVID-19 to enable continuity. The Anti-Amyloid Treatment in Asymptomatic Alzheimer's Disease (A4) trial was a phase III clinical trial evaluating the efficacy and safety of solanezumab in preclinical Alzheimer's disease. Due to social distancing measures implemented during the COVID-19 pandemic, mobile research nurses were deployed to conduct home visits and administer trial infusions every month. Initiated in 2014, this trial did not originally include home visits in the trial protocol but were added in 2020. Due to this implementation, active A4 participants were offered the option to continue receiving investigational products [25]. Another landmark DCT was conducted by Boehringer Ingelheim for the treatment of major depressive disorder in a registrational phase II trial. These approaches will be discussed in more depth in Chap. 3: Regulatory Landscape and Chap. 4: Methodology and Protocol Development.

In a survey from 127 senior clinical research executives from September through October 2021, 77% of respondents planned to run a hybrid DCT within the next 12 months, compared to 59% for the previous year [26]. Regulators and health authorities all over the world recognize that DCT approaches have the potential to improve accessibility, diversity, and retention in clinical trials [12, 27]. They will not be appropriate for every trial and the key opportunities are reduced participant and caregiver burden, which would facilitate the participation of underserved participants. Data collected by DCTs tend to be more representative of the real world, which has always been a limitation in historical clinical trial data applicability. Key challenges to be addressed are investigator oversight and participant safety when face-to-face contact is limited, which is why hybrid trials may be more suitable in the immediate implementation term.

Quiz Questions
1. All of the following are cited as reasons for the evolving need for DCTs, EXCEPT:
   (A) Need for participant-centric trials and shift in regulatory attention for diversity and inclusion
   (B) Lack of geographic accessibility for participants
   (C) Participant preference to control treatment choice in a clinical trial
   (D) Slow clinical trial recruitment rate leading to premature clinical trial termination
2. Which is an example of notable industry partnership in DCTs?
   (A) Walmart and Medable
   (B) Thread and Amazon
   (C) Thread and Walgreens
   (D) CVS and Walgreens
3. DCTs typically encompass which of the following digital health components?
   (A) Telehealth, digital therapeutics, mobile health
   (B) Telehealth, artificial intelligence, remote assessments, mobile health
   (C) Telehealth, remote assessments, health information technology
   (D) Telehealth, health information technology, mobile health
4. True or False: Eli Lilly and Genentech were the first two companies prior to the COVID-19 pandemic to pilot DCTs in non-oncology participants.

Answers to Quiz Questions
1. C
2. B
3. D
4. False—Eli Lilly and Pfizer were the first companies to pilot DCTs in erectile dysfunction and overactive bladder, respectively.

Bibliography

1. Unger JM, Cook E, Tai E, Bleyer A. The role of clinical trial participation in cancer Research: barriers, evidence, and strategies. Am Soc Clin Oncol Educ Book Am Soc Clin Oncol Annu Meet. 2016;35:185–98. https://doi.org/10.1200/EDBK_156686.
2. Desai M. Recruitment and retention of participants in clinical studies: critical issues and challenges. Perspect Clin Res. 2020;11(2):51–3. https://doi.org/10.4103/picr.PICR_6_20.
3. Nipp RD, Hong K, Paskett ED. Overcoming barriers to clinical trial enrollment. Am Soc Clin Oncol Educ Book. 2019;39:105–14. https://doi.org/10.1200/EDBK_243729.
4. CISCRP Perceptions and insights study 2021; 2021.
5. Unger JM, Hershman DL, Till C, et al. "When offered to participate": a systematic review and meta-analysis of patient agreement to participate in cancer clinical trials. JNCI J Natl Cancer Inst. 2021;113(3):244–57. https://doi.org/10.1093/jnci/djaa155.
6. National Cancer Institute. Clinical trial participation among US adults. 2022.
7. Carlisle B, Kimmelman J, Ramsay T, MacKinnon N. Unsuccessful trial accrual and human subjects protections: an empirical analysis of recently closed trials. Clin Trials Lond Engl. 2015;12(1):77–83. https://doi.org/10.1177/1740774514558307.
8. Research C for DE and Patient-Focused Drug Development: Collecting Comprehensive and Representative Input. 2021. https://www.fda.gov/regulatory-information/search-fda-guidance-documents/patient-focused-drug-development-collecting-comprehensive-and-representative-input. Accessed 9 Dec 2023.

9. Research C for DE and Enhancing the Diversity of Clinical Trial Populations—Eligibility Criteria, Enrollment Practices, and Trial Designs Guidance for Industry. 2020. https://www.fda.gov/regulatory-information/search-fda-guidance-documents/enhancing-diversity-clinical-trial-populations-eligibility-criteria-enrollment-practices-and-trial. Accessed 9 Dec 2023.
10. Andino JJ, Zhu Z, Surapaneni M, Dunn RL, Ellimoottil C. Interstate telehealth use by Medicare beneficiaries before and after COVID-19 licensure waivers, 2017–2020. Health Aff (Millwood). 2022;41(6):838–45. https://doi.org/10.1377/hlthaff.2021.01825.
11. Xue JZ, Smietana K, Poda P, Webster K, Yang G, Agrawal G. Clinical trial recovery from COVID-19 disruption. Nat Rev Drug Discov. 2020;19(10):662–3. https://doi.org/10.1038/d41573-020-00150-9.
12. Research C for DE and Decentralized Clinical Trials for Drugs, Biological Products, and Devices. 2023. https://www.fda.gov/regulatory-information/search-fda-guidance-documents/decentralized-clinical-trials-drugs-biological-products-and-devices. Accessed 9 Dec 2023.
13. Lin CC, Bruinooge SS, Kirkwood MK, et al. Association between geographic access to cancer care, insurance, and receipt of chemotherapy: geographic distribution of oncologists and travel distance. J Clin Oncol. 2015;33(28):3177–85. https://doi.org/10.1200/JCO.2015.61.1558.
14. Lindsay AA, Cooper JA. Is this an interventional clinical trial or observational study? How- and why—it is important to write protocols that make this distinction clear. WCG Published July 24, 2018. https://www.wcg-clinical.com/insights/is-this-an-interventional-clinical-trial-or-observational-study-how-and-why-it-is-important-to-write-protocols-that-make-this-distinction-clear/. Accessed 9 Dec 2023.
15. Thadhani R. Formal trials versus observational studies. In: Mehta A, Beck M, Sunder-Plassmann G, editors. Fabry disease: perspectives from 5 years of FOS. Oxford PharmaGenesis; 2006. http://www.ncbi.nlm.nih.gov/books/NBK11597/.
16. What Are Clinical Trials and Studies? | National Institute on Aging. https://www.nia.nih.gov/health/clinical-trials-and-studies/what-are-clinical-trials-and-studies. Accessed 9 Dec 2023.
17. DIGITAL HEALTH TRIALS.
18. trialshome. About DCTs—Trials@Home. 2019. https://trialsathome.com/about-rdcts/. Accessed 9 Dec 2023.
19. FDA and Duke Launch Public-Private Partnership to Modernize Clinical Trials.
20. Eilenberg KL, Hoover AM, Rutherford ML, Melfi CA, Segal S. From informed consent through database lock: an interactive clinical trial conducted using the internet. Drug Inf J. 2004;38(3):239–51. https://doi.org/10.1177/009286150403800303.

21. Pfizer Conducts First "Virtual" Clinical Trial Allowing Patients to Participate Regardless Of Geography | Pfizer. https://www.pfizer.com/news/press-release/press-release-detail/pfizer_conducts_first_virtual_clinical_trial_allowing_patients_to_participate_regardless_of_geography. Accessed 9 Dec 2023.
22. Orri M, Lipset CH, Jacobs BP, Costello AJ, Cummings SR. Web-based trial to evaluate the efficacy and safety of tolterodine ER 4mg in participants with overactive bladder: REMOTE trial. Contemp Clin Trials. 2014;38(2):190–7. https://doi.org/10.1016/j.cct.2014.04.009.
23. Adams DV, Long S, Fleury ME. Association of remote technology use and other decentralization tools with patient likelihood to enroll in cancer clinical trials. JAMA Netw Open. 2022;5(7):e2220053. https://doi.org/10.1001/jamanetworkopen.2022.20053.
24. Childers L. Decentralized Clinical Trials: Bringing Care Directly to Patients. 2022;16. https://www.oncnursingnews.com/view/decentralized-clinical-trials-bringing-care-directly-to-patients. Accessed 9 Dec 2023.
25. Challenging Global Alzheimer's Study Involving Home Infusions Exceeds Expectations. https://www.clinicalleader.com/doc/challenging-global-alzheimer-s-study-involving-home-infusions-exceeds-expectations-0001. Accessed 9 Dec 2023.
26. LaHucik K. About 77% of clinical research execs expect to run decentralized trials in next 12 months: survey. Fierce Biotech Published November 17, 2021. https://www.fiercebiotech.com/cro/nearly-80-clinical-research-execs-expect-to-run-decentralized-trials-next-12-months-survey. Accessed 9 Dec 2023.
27. De Jong AJ, Van Rijssel TI, Zuidgeest MGP, et al. Opportunities and challenges for decentralized clinical trials: European regulators' perspective. Clin Pharmacol Ther. 2022;112(2):344–52. https://doi.org/10.1002/cpt.2628.

Technology Landscape and Requirements

Anna H. Yang and Isaac R. Rodriguez-Chavez

Objectives
By the end of this chapter, you will be able to:

1. Understand the data flow between systems and vendors during a clinical trial.
2. Define health data interoperability and describe US-based policy efforts to harmonize adoption.
3. Describe technology implementation considerations in a DCT.
4. List predictions and future trends for emerging cross-industry trends.

A. H. Yang (✉)
Genentech, A Member of the Roche Group,
South San Francisco, CA, USA

I. R. Rodriguez-Chavez
CEO & Principal Independent Consultant, Scientific, Clinical, Regulatory Affairs and Digital Health Technologies, 4Biosolutions Consulting, Rockville, MD, USA

© The Author(s), under exclusive license to Springer Nature Switzerland AG 2024
A. H. Yang, I. R. Rodriguez-Chavez (eds.), *Fundamentals of Decentralized Clinical Trials*,
https://doi.org/10.1007/978-3-031-62877-1_2

Data Flow Between Systems in a Clinical Trial

Introduction to Findable, Accessible, Interoperable and Reusable Data Principles

In 2016, a diverse group of stakeholders from academic, industry, funding agencies, non-for-profit organizations and scholarly publishers designed and jointly endorsed a set of concise and measurable data principles known as the Findable, Accessible, Interoperable and Reusable (FAIR) principles. FAIR data principles were established as a solution to improve the infrastructure supporting the reuse of scholarly data (e.g., scientific research data) and metadata (e.g., associated metadata, analytical models and algorithms, analytical provenance, and ontologies and standards). In this manner, data can be easily findable and reused across the field and encourage good data management as the key conduit that leads to knowledge discovery and innovation.

In short, FAIR principles state that data should also be made Findable, Accessible, Interoperable and Reusable (FAIR) [1]. Regarding associated metadata, it refers to data sets that describe research data that explain the methodology, instruments, variables, and technical specifications to facilitate reuse. Findable means that it should be easy for humans and computers to find the information; there should be metadata that exists for users to find that data. Accessible means that once the data and metadata are found, the user should be able to obtain the data and metadata, whether through open-access, authentication, authorization, etc. Interoperable means that the data must share a common structure; metadata use must also be recognized. Reusable means that the data should be well-described to be combined in different settings [1].

Applying the FAIR Principles in the Context of a Clinical Trial

In a traditional clinical trial, there are multiple systems and vendors involved in the collection, management, and analysis of the data and metadata. There are common systems that are typically involved, including:

2 Technology Landscape and Requirements

- Electronic Data Capture (EDC): The EDC system is the primary system used to collect data in a clinical study. It may be hosted by a third-party vendor and managed by a Sponsor. Trial personnel will enter data directly into the system, and the EDC may be used to generate study reports and provide an overview of the data quality.
- Clinical Trial Management System (CTMS): The CTMS is used to manage high-level summary information and conduct of the trial. This includes tracking study progress, study timelines, study budget, and study investigator information. CTMS may be used to generate reports on study performance and milestones.
- Laboratory Information Management System (LIMS): The LIMS is used to manage laboratory data, including biospecimen tracking, test results, and quality control data. The LIMS may be integrated with—or connected with—the EDC system, which allows for seamless transfer of lab data.
- Randomization and Blinding System (RBS): This system is designed specifically for randomization and blinding the study subjects to ensure a completely randomized and unbiased approach. This system is also hosted by a third-party vendor and may be integrated with the EDC system.
- Data Management System (DMS): A system used to collect, manage, and clean the data and may be integrated with EDC.
- Statistical Analysis System (SAS): A system used to analyze the data and may be integrated with EDC.
- Safety Reporting System (SRS): A system used to manage adverse event reporting during a trial and may be integrated with EDC.
- Electronic Health Record (EHR): A software system that is used to store and manage participant health information electronically. It helps to ensure that the data is accurate, complete, and accessible.
- Electronic Patient Reported Outcomes (ePRO): A digital collection of trial participant-reported outcomes using standards-based question banks. It maintains a link between patient-reported data and interpretations aiding provenance tracking.

- Ontology Management Systems (OMS): House-controlled clinical terminologies helping standardize annotations. It maintains references to external ontologies aiding discoverability.
- Data Warehouses and Repositories (DWRs): Centralized databases to store, standardize and integrate research data assets. They support consistent metadata schemas and data dictionaries.
  - Clinical Trial Data Warehouse (CTDWH): CTDWH is a software system that is used to store and manage clinical trial data. It helps to ensure that the data is secure, accessible, and reusable.
- Workflow Management Systems (WMS): Systems that automate and track Data Management System (DMS) sequencing of data processes maintaining provenance. It ensures use of standardized terminologies and ontologies.
- Cloud Computing Platforms (CCP): Platforms that facilitate scalable and accessible data and analytics pipelines. Provide infrastructure for FAIR data sharing through public Application Programming Interfaces (APIs).
- Analytics Platforms (APs): Trace data from collection to statistical Data Management System (DMS)analysis output for transparent provenance. Apply FAIR principles to analytic scripts and metadata enabling reproducibility.
- Container Technologies (CTs Dockers): Package data analytical pipelines with dependencies improving reproducibility. Maintain lineage between data, scripts, parameters, and outputs.
- Metadata Catalogs (MCs): Index and maintain searchable metadata enabling discoverability. Map local metadata to global ontologies aiding interoperability.
  - Metadata Repository (MDR): MDR is a software system that is used to store and manage metadata. It helps to ensure that the metadata is well-documented, organized, and reusable.
- Unique and Persistent Identifiers (UPIs): Assign digital object identifiers to datasets, algorithms and other digital research outputs that persist over time for citation and access.

- Semantic Web Technologies (SWTs): Annotate data assets using World Wide Web Consortium (W3C) standards like RDF making data interpretable by the computer. Map local terminologies to common ontologies through Resource Description Framework (RDF) schema.

Data may flow between these systems in various ways, through manual deliveries or automation. For example, data may be entered directly into the EDC by study personnel or automatically transferred from LIMS. Data may also be exported from one system and imported into another for analysis or reporting purposes. It is important for all systems and vendors to work together to ensure that the data is collected, managed, and analyzed in a consistent and accurate manner.

In a DCT, it is essential to establish a dataflow management plan to map out the end-to-end flow of the origin of data to the destination of the data. Due to the increased complexities of systems and vendors managed by the CRO and/or study team, a solid understanding of each data source and its link to subsequent data sources is critical. This applies to each individual team member, rather than just the data management delivery teammates.

Health Data Interoperability and US-Based Efforts to Harmonize Adoption

Data privacy and security standards that affect clinical trial conduct have evolved over time in response to changing policies. In 1996, The Health Insurance Portability and Accountability Act (HIPAA) established privacy and security standards for protected health information (PHI). HIPAA was created to protect PHI and applied to clinical trials because of the need to protect participant data [2]. In 1996, The International Conference on Harmonization (ICH) Guidelines for Good Clinical Practice (GCP) E6(R3) also created a unified standard for clinical trial design, conduct, monitoring, and reporting to ensure the protection of study participants' rights, safety, and wellbeing [3]. It also requires confidentiality of personal data.

To explain health data interoperability, imagine we are trying to navigate from Point A, located in New Jersey, to Point B, located in California. We would use the highway systems to travel across the nation, interfacing with highways and all sorts of local roads. Regardless of the terrain or sizes of the towns along the way, the road infrastructure enables us to get to our destination. Imagine if there did not exist a highway system to connect all the local towns, how difficult it would be to navigate our way. This is the problem we faced and continue to face today in the United States' healthcare information system. There is an urgent need to transform local health information into secure, integrated, and interoperable networks in compliance with regulatory requirements and following best practices for technical standards [4].

In 2004, President George W. Bush signed Executive Order 13335, creating the Office of the National Coordinator (ONC) for Health Information Technology in the Department of Health and Human Services (HHS). In 2009, the ONC was codified in legislation with the enactment of the Health Information Technology for Economic and Clinical Health (HITECH) Act, part of the American Recovery and Reinvestment Act. While ONC is not able to mandate any health interoperability standards, HITECH provided short-term funding to HHS to create an incentive program in which certain eligible professionals and hospitals received payment for adopting and using electronic health records (EHRs) technology. HITECH also gave ONC the permanent authority to promote the widespread adoption of standardized and certified EHR technology, facilitate the secure use and exchange of interoperable health information, and promote the delivery of safe, efficient, cost-effective high-quality care. In essence, ONC does not enforce any health data standards, but the incentive payment program helped drive their authority and thus, widespread adoption of standard health information exchange. Between 2008 to 2015, the health field saw a dramatic rise in EHR technology adoption. Adoption of basic EHR technology for office-based physicians grew from 17 to 58% and non-federal acute hospitals grew from 9 to 84% [5].

More recently, in October 2023, President Biden issued an Executive Order focused on Safe, Secure, and Trustworthy Artificial Intelligence (White House, 2023, October 30) [6]. The order aims to ensure America's leadership in harnessing AI's potential and managing its risks, particularly in healthcare and clinical research. It establishes new standards for AI safety and security, safeguarding privacy, promoting equity, and advancing innovation. Key directives include:

1. Requiring developers of powerful AI systems to share safety test results and critical information with the U.S. government.
2. Developing standards, tools, and tests to ensure AI systems are safe, secure, and trustworthy.
3. Setting strong standards for screening against risks of using AI in engineering dangerous biological materials.

Furthermore, the order underscores AI's significance in healthcare and clinical research, directing actions to:

1. Create a framework fostering AI innovation while protecting participant safety, privacy, and ensuring fair access to its benefits.
2. Establish a working group to devise a plan for AI's use in healthcare and clinical research.

This order aligns with the Biden-Harris Administration's strategy for responsible innovation and builds on prior efforts, including securing commitments from 15 leading companies for the safe, secure, and trustworthy development of AI. It is expected that this new executive order will enhance the interoperability and technical standards applied to novel technologies used in clinical research and healthcare.

Interoperability is defined as the ability of different information systems, devices and applications (systems) to access, exchange, integrate and cooperatively use data in a coordinated manner, within and across organizational, regional and national boundaries, to provide timely and seamless portability of information and optimize the health of individuals [7]. Interoperability enables different sources of information to be exchanged and then used to make clinical decisions. For example, health data from the physician's electronic health record should be able to be shared quickly with all members of the health team, including trial participants. All the information coming from trial participants' records should be able to fit together. Loosely applied, interoperability can be thought of as a cell phone network, in which it doesn't matter where the call is originating from, where the recipient is located, which brand of cell phone, what cell network provider it is, the call will go through. Applied to healthcare, health data interoperability enables all types of health information to connect to each other, through standardized approaches, and can increase clinical safety, promote health equity, and speed up public health emergency responses.

Clear data standards are important to ensure health data interoperability. ONC works with the industry, public entities, and trial participants to define and certify these standards. The ONC set up the United States Core Data for Interoperability (US CDI). USCDI includes data classes such as allergies and intolerances, clinical notes, problem list, health insurance information, vital signs, or laboratory results. USCDI are the minimum dataset that is required to be supported by an EHR. There is also a recent USCDI+ initiative that includes additional data standard components beyond routine clinical care; the USCDI+ initiative is an extension of USCDI for clinical trials data element research standards. In addition, on the frontier of health data information exchange, the ONC established the Trusted Exchange Framework and Common Agreement network (TEFCA), which is a common set of principles, terms, and conditions to support the development of a Common Agreement that would help enable nationwide exchange of electronic health information (EHI) across disparate health information networks. (HINs). TEFCA aims to expedite the sharing of EHI across networks, healthcare providers, health plans, and individuals.

Technology Implementation Considerations

When implementing technology in a clinical trial, some key considerations include:

1. Legal data privacy and security: Trial participant data is highly sensitive, and it is important to ensure that all data is stored securely, with access limited to authorized personnel only. Thus, it is required to comply with local laws on this topic.
2. Regulatory compliance: Clinical trials are subject to a range of regulations across regulatory jurisdictions where they are conducted, and it is required to ensure that all technology used in the trial complies with these regulations.
3. System compatibility: The technology used in the trial must be compatible with existing digital systems used by the trial team and other stakeholders, such as electronic health records (EHRs).
4. User experience: The technology should be easy to use and accessible to all users, including trial participants, trial coordinators, and healthcare providers.
5. Reliability and accuracy: The technology used in the trial must be reliable and accurate, with minimal risk of data loss or errors.
6. Data integration: The technology used should be capable of integrating data from multiple digital sources, such as DHTs and other medical devices, to provide a comprehensive view of trial participant's health.
7. Scalability: The technology used should be scalable to accommodate changes in the size and scope of the trial, as well as future trials.
8. Cost-effectiveness: The technology used should be cost-effective, with a clear return on investment and minimal impact on the overall budget for the trial.

When a clinical research team assesses which technology partners to bring into the study, they consider multitude factors. The first consideration is: what is the target digital clinical data that the team wants to collect? Let's walk through an example.

Question/consideration	Impact on study execution
Track a trial participant's symptoms—subjective	Use a validated questionnaire
Track trial participant's symptoms—objective	Collect biometric measures using DHTs
Use a trial participant-facing platform to collect data	Ensure the privacy, security, and integrity of data collected
Long-term tracking/follow-up	Consider using data tokenization
Virtual participant recruitment	Consider using electronic health records, claims, or data tokenization

Technology Components

Many DCT platform companies offer some type of "trial hub", a dashboard that offers telehealth, clinical trial status, some level of trial participant reported information, and digital communication that may or may not include alerts. The dashboard is offered as a portal or website application (web app) for the site with a unique login identification (ID). The dashboard may have user-specific firewalls, for example, an Investigator or sub-Investigator would be able to dial into the telehealth appointment, but the research coordinators would only be able to view the appointment details and not dial into the appointment. These customized firewalls are not always broadly offered, and it is important for the study team to critically assess the platform's capabilities.

> *Study team tip*: Some questions you can ask the technology vendor as you evaluate their offerings and capabilities are: Does your dashboard offer customizable roles and responsibilities depending on the user (investigator, coordinator, pharmacist)? Is there a way to communicate between trial team personnel on the dashboard, ie; if a dose needs to be held or modified? Can the dashboard act as an eSource for the DCT (source of truth for official trial documentation records)?

For telehealth, some vendor platforms offer their own in-house videoconferencing technology. Others may choose to outsource to another third party, such as Microsoft Teams. Study teams should plan for additional time and people resources to conduct technology assessments, as each clinical trial site may need to submit the platform through their internal privacy and security reviews, and newer telehealth platforms may only slow down the process. Data integrations across multiple platforms that do not communicate and must be manually cleaned can slow down DCT implementation.

> *Aspiration point*: If the clinical trial site is an early adopter of health technology and flexible, try to assess if you can integrate with the health system's own telehealth system and/or electronic trial participant reported portal. This way, participants and sites can see more seamless embedding of their routine clinical practice and DCT-related activities. This is the ultimate goal of clinical research, after all, which is to provide the gold standard of medical care to all participants and not burden researchers with additional trial-specific tasks. If using an EDC system, try to pick a system that has improved data integration with other clinical technologies and direct data capture.

Clinical trial status may include total participant enrollment (x out of y trial participants needed to complete a DCT), participants currently on treatment (participants who are still taking the medication), participants who have completed treatment (in the follow-up period), participants lost to follow-up, withdrawn/dropped out participants. It is important to note that the Clinical Trial Management System (CTMS) will likely remain the source of truth for all trial metrics mentioned above. This portion of the dashboard's purpose is to provide broad awareness for the study team, particularly a decentralized study that may involve multiple sites.

> *Aspiration point*: Particularly in DCT studies, we have the unique ability to offer specialized clinical oversight to trial participants who may not have had access previously. For example, a lung cancer participant with a rare mutation who lives in a rural setting needed to drive 100 miles to an academic site. The participant is prescribed with an oral medication, which can be shipped directly to his or her home. To decrease the burden needed to travel to and from the academic site every month, the participant can be seen locally by his or her general oncologist as well as through telehealth with a lung cancer specialist. This specialist knows which questions to ask and symptoms to closely monitor for; the local oncologist can be invited to the telehealth appointments and follow-up with CT scans or laboratory tests as appropriate. In this manner, trial participants receive appropriate care regardless of their location and the local oncologist can maintain a relationship with the trial participant while gaining insight into how to manage a rare tumor type.

Trial participant-reported information is a broad category that may include eCOA, eDiary, and digital devices containing biometric data. eCOA vendors are vast due to the nature that each eCOA instrument needs to be validated down to the type of questions and user interface. Many DCT platforms will outsource their eCOA because of this. eDiary is a way to digitally track a trial participant's medication adherence and may likely not be the eSource of participant drug intake, due to the validity of participant-inputted data. eDiary also includes Direct-to-Participant (DtP) shipment. DtP includes mostly oral medications but can also include parenteral medications that can be given in the home with proper oversight. A few companies offer smart digital medication tracking and herein lies the opportunity to integrate a DCT platform with this capability. For digital devices, this includes DHTs (wellness and medical grade) and basic medical devices that capture vitals (blood pressure, scales). Once these digital devices are used in a setting outside of the clinic, the diagnostic potential becomes variable. Despite the skepticism, these digital devices remain an area of immense opportunity for decentralized, at-home clinical research.

Digital communication is a way for trial participants to communicate with their research team, either for study-related or technology-related questions. Some technology platforms offer a chatbot, a conversational tool using generative artificial intelligence that has a database of frequently asked questions that can triage questions for nurses or digital navigators. If there is a free-text field, it is critical to put in place a mitigation plan for adverse event (AE) reporting and protected health information (PHI) exposure.

> *Study team tip*: Alerts are a somewhat controversial topic for DCT platforms. While a nice-to-have, the concern is a legal one. If the study team needs to alert the trial participant (or if the participant needs to alert the study team) and the information is not relayed quickly, who is responsible? The sponsor holds the IND and therefore is accountable for all study events, but the platform needs to assume responsibility as well and a mitigation plan clearly mapped out. If this process is not clearly defined or there is risk of study personnel turnover and therefore risk for inadequate training, a word of advice: Stick to traditional processes of placing the alert responsibility on study teams and approved sponsor-delegates (CROs).

List Predictions and Future Trends for Emerging Cross-Industry Trends

DCTs have really gained momentum in recent years, particularly due to the COVID-19 pandemic. The intersection of health and technology may continue to bring forth notable foreseeable trends, such as:

- Linking of EHRs: Some DCT platforms are starting to boast access to EHR data, which would greatly accelerate participant recruitment speed, completeness of data capture, and even database lock timelines. There is an emerging concept of tokenization in which trial participants' data can remain anonymized and tracked longitudinally.
- Digital health technology (DHT) measurements as endpoints: traditional clinical endpoints may be captured digitally and accepted for regulatory submission. DHTs yield clinical laboratory measurements (continuous glucose monitoring, pulse oximetry), functional measurements (heart rate, respiratory rate, temperature, weight, seizures, syncope), and psychological/emotional/behavioral measurements (anxiety, depression, mood, excitement) that can be captured, analyzed, reported and stored digitally.
- Artificial intelligence (AI) and machine learning (ML): The ability to collect and analyze large amounts of data is becoming increasingly important. Advanced analytics can help identify patterns and trends that would be otherwise difficult to detect using traditional methods. With AI/ML, researchers have the ability to analyze the data more efficiently and accurately. AI/ML can also be used to develop predictive models that can help identify trial participants at risk for developing adverse events, medication noncompliance, and potentially disease progression. Digital patient twins are being evaluated as a model for predicting trial participants' individual disease journeys.
- Expansion of the Digiverse in DCTs: A major trend in DCTs is the increased adoption of innovative technologies and DHTs to enable these investigations across therapeutic areas. Thus, the digiverse is understood as the digital universe of solutions that are carefully designed and implemented for each DCT and that represent the digital technology ecosystem that is customized for each trial. The digiverse for each DCT represents a digital hallmark or print that defines that unique technology ecosystem used for a particular DCT and it needs to account for

national and global scalability. Thus, a DCT may include from one to as many digital technological components as needed to support specific trial-related activities. The more the number of technologies and DHTs used in a DCT, the more complex the digiverse of that trial is and vice versa [8]. Advantages of designing and implementing a digiverse in a DCT are the same as originally described for DCTs in general.

Quiz Questions
1. Which of the following is true about the FAIR data principles?
    (I) FAIR stands for: Findable, Accessible, Interoperable, and Reusable
    (II) A group of academics, industry, funding agencies, and scholarly publishers designed and endorsed the standards together
    (III) Accessible means that both the data and metadata are able to be retrieved through a log-in
    (A) I, II
    (B) I, II, and III
    (C) II, III
    (D) I only
2. Which of the following ACCURATELY describes CTMS?
    (A) Used to manage high-level summary information and conduct of the trial. This includes tracking study progress, study timelines, study budget, and study investigator information
    (B) Is the primary system used to collected data in a clinical study
    (C) Used to manage laboratory data, including biospecimen tracking, test results, and quality control data
    (D) A system used to analyze the data and may be integrated with EDC

3. What is the term used to describe this technology implementation consideration? "The technology used should be scalable to accommodate changes in the size and scope of the trial, as well as future trials."
   (A) Data privacy and security
   (B) System compatibility
   (C) Data integration
   (D) Scalability
4. Thinking ahead, what is one way for pharmaceutical companies to greatly speed up participant recruitment using DCTs?
   (A) Hybrid registrational phase III trials
   (B) Linking of EHRs
   (C) Digital health technologies
   (D) Telehealth

Answers to Quiz Questions
1. B
2. A
3. D
4. B

Bibliography

1. Wilkinson MD, Dumontier M, Aalbersberg IJJ, et al. The FAIR guiding principles for scientific data management and stewardship. Sci Data. 2016;3(1):160018. https://doi.org/10.1038/sdata.2016.18.
2. Health Insurance Portability and Accountability Act of 1996. ASPE Published August 20, 1996. https://aspe.hhs.gov/reports/health-insurance-portability-accountability-act-1996. Accessed 9 Dec 2023.
3. ICH_E6(R3)_DraftGuideline_2023_0519.pdf. https://database.ich.org/sites/default/files/ICH_E6%28R3%29_DraftGuideline_2023_0519.pdf. Accessed 9 Dec 2023.

4. The Path To Interoperability—YouTube. https://www.youtube.com/watch?v=PaWcU7rqqyA. Accessed 9 Dec 2023.
5. onc_cj_2018_final.pdf. https://www.healthit.gov/sites/default/files/onc_cj_2018_final.pdf. Accessed 9 Dec 2023.
6. House TW. Executive order on the safe, secure, and trustworthy development and use of artificial intelligence. The White House Published October 30, 2023. https://www.whitehouse.gov/briefing-room/presidential-actions/2023/10/30/executive-order-on-the-safe-secure-and-trustworthy-development-and-use-of-artificial-intelligence/. Accessed 9 Dec 2023.
7. IF12352.pdf. https://crsreports.congress.gov/product/pdf/IF/IF12352. Accessed 9 Dec 2023.
8. Rodriguez-Chavez IR. ICT May 2022. calameo.com. https://www.calameo.com/read/00611338552c319d1b027?page=54. Accessed 9 Dec 2023.

Regulatory Landscape

Isaac R. Rodriguez-Chavez
and Anna H. Yang

Objectives
By the end of this chapter, you will be able to:

1. Describe the regulatory stage pre-COVID-19 pandemic.
2. List regulatory adjustments during the COVID-19 pandemic.
3. Summarize the FDA Draft DCT Guidance released in 2023.

Regulatory Stage Pre COVID-19 Pandemic

Prior to the COVID-19 pandemic, the regulatory framework for decentralized clinical trials (DCTs) was forming. FDA had released guidance in 1997 around electronic signature capture. In

---

I. R. Rodriguez-Chavez
CEO & Principal Independent Consultant, Scientific, Clinical, Regulatory Affairs and Digital Health Technologies, 4Biosolutions Consulting, Rockville, MD, USA

A. H. Yang (✉)
Genentech, A Member of the Roche Group,
South San Francisco, CA, USA

2007, FDA issued final guidance on Computerized Systems Used in Clinical Investigations. In 2013, FDA published final guidance around Electronic Source Data in Clinical Investigations followed by another final guidance in 2016 related to Use of Electronic Informed Consent, Questions and Answers.

In 2016, Congress passed the twenty-first Century Cures Act to facilitate novel trial designs and the use of other data sources to support FDA approval. The goal was to accelerate medical product development to trial participants more quickly and efficiently. Some changes to modernize clinical trial design include utilizing clinical outcome assessments (COA), digital endpoints, digital health technologies (DHTs), digital technologies and real-world evidence. This encouraged the industry to adopt a wider pool of data sources and set the stage for implementing decentralized approaches to collect evidence during a clinical trial. Furthermore, it balanced the need for increased privacy protection with the increase of data sharing, a theme that continues to be central to the field of clinical research using DCT approaches enabled by DHTs.

Telemedicine as part of telehealth and videoconferencing with patients was established in some large health systems for routine follow-up purposes. These virtual visits were largely unexplored in the context of interventional trials. In the US, the FDA recognized the large and persistent data gap that separated important scientific advances and the technologies needed to translate those advances into new therapies for trial participants and new ways to protect public health. Therefore in 2019, the FDA Technology Modernization Action Plan (TMAP) was established to modernize the use of technology at FDA.

The Consolidated Appropriations Act of 2022 incorporated numerous measures centered on advancing healthcare inclusivity, diversity, and technological innovation [1]. Specifically, the Act addresses DCTs, equity diversity, and inclusion (EDI), and DHTs to enhance healthcare outcomes and foster progress in clinical research.

In relation to DCTs, the Act mandates the FDA to provide guidance to enhance diversity within clinical trials, encourage the adoption of DCTs, and assess the appropriate utilization of DHTs in these trials. This guidance aims to encompass considerations for DCTs, focusing on engaging, enrolling, and retaining a diverse clinical population that reflects various facets such as race, ethnicity, age, gender, and geographic location, as applicable. Moreover, the FDA is tasked with ensuring that trial sponsors establish specific diversity-oriented objectives and tactics for both participant recruitment and training of clinical personnel.

Concerning EDI, the Act allocates funding for diverse programs and initiatives across sectors like education, healthcare, and housing, aiming to promote and support equity, diversity, and inclusion efforts.

Additionally, the Act includes provisions concerning DHTs, offering financial support for research and development in this domain and fostering initiatives to encourage their application in healthcare and clinical research endeavors.

Similarly, the Food and Drug Omnibus Reform Act of 2022 (FDORA) enacted major changes to federal regulations governing clinical trials [2]. Key focus areas included promoting diversity in clinical trials, improving enrollment diversity and inclusion, and expanding adoption of DHTs.

Regarding DCTs, FDORA mandated the Department of Health and Human Services (HHS) Secretary to provide guidance on diversifying trial populations. This aims to facilitate meaningful engagement, enrollment, and retention of diverse participants based on factors like race, ethnicity, age, gender, and location.

For EDI, FDORA required sponsors of late-phase drug and certain device trials to submit diversity action plans outlining enrollment goals, rationale, and strategies for recruiting diverse groups. However, the HHS Secretary can waive this mandate during public health emergencies or other extenuating circumstances.

To promote DHTs, FDORA compelled the HHS Secretary to issue updated guidance on integrating digital tools into trials and enabling innovative study designs. It also prioritized global alignment by directing collaboration with international regulators to harmonize regulations and best practices for DCTs, EDI, and DHT adoption across geographies.

In short, the Act established new standards and directives focused on diversifying clinical trial participant populations, removing representation barriers, and incorporating emerging

DHTs—ultimately aiming to enhance EDI, and technological innovation across clinical research.

Regulatory Adjustments During the COVID-19 Pandemic

In a short period of time in late 2019 to the early months of 2020, the localized outbreak of COVID-19 erupted into a global pandemic that strained even the most resilient health systems. Governments and health systems deployed several strategies to limit transmission, protect the capacity of health systems, and prioritize the resourcing of front-line healthcare workers [3]. Innovative solutions that increase the clinical care capacity were required to substantially reconfigure existing health facilities and repurpose existing public and private facilities for acute health care management, and this was seen in remote and low-resource areas as well. This applied to the continuity of clinical trials to save trial participant lives, in which recruitment, enrollment, follow-up and monitoring participants, outcome measures, and delivery and administration of (investigational) drugs and devices faced challenges, and continuing such trials were an ethical and moral imperative [4].

Many trial leaders converted trial activities from in-person to virtual settings. A cross-sectional, exploratory survey on the uptake of decentralized approaches in the early phase of the pandemic. The Trials@Home Initiative in Europe conducted a survey in 18 member organizations (CROs = 2, pharmaceutical companies = 9, research networks = 2, technology companies = 3, universities = 2). First, almost all the organizations (n = 16) had to put a proportion of their trials on hold, mainly due to safety concerns for participants and staff, followed by closure of facilities due to lockdown measures, restriction of in-person assessments, and avoiding unnecessary exposure. Seventeen organizations reported that a proportion of their existing trials did not change due to COVID-19, due to the existing flexible nature of their trial

3 Regulatory Landscape

protocols. Sixteen organizations reported that for trials that did not have existing flexible natures, they implemented DCT modifications, such as reviewing photos of diagnostics instead of in-person visits, trial set-up and design, intervention and follow-up, operations and coordination and other trial activities [4]. There were a few modifications that rose in implementation popularity compared to prior to COVID-19. They were participant-health care provider interaction and communication, direct-to-participant IMP supply, clinic visits changed to telehealth visits, and source document verification.

In the wake of the clinical trial disruption and to help trial sponsors during these uncertain times, health authorities from the FDA and European Medicines Agency (EMA) provided emergency guidance. From 2020 through 2022, FDA issued 84 new guidance documents to provide policies, transparency, and flexibility, as appropriate, to address vital medical products for COVID-19 and the public health issues facing the U.S. during this pandemic. In September 2020, the FDA also launched the Digital Health Center of Excellence to empower stakeholders to advance health care by fostering responsible and high-quality digital health innovation [5].

During and after the main waves of COVID-19 and as of late 2023, FDA has continued to expand the regulatory framework for DCTs by issuing the following guidance documents: "Enhancing the Diversity of Clinical Trial Populations, Eligibility Criteria, Enrollment Practices, and Trial Designs" (final guidance, 2020); "Digital Health Technologies for Remote Data Acquisition in Clinical Investigations" (draft guidance, 2021); "Clinical Decision Support Software" (final guidance, 2022); "Diversity Plans to Improve Enrollment of Participants from Underrepresented Racial and Ethnic Populations in Clinical Trials" (final guidance, 2022); and the "Decentralized Clinical Trials for Drugs, Biological Products, and Devices" draft guidance of 2023 previously mentioned. Similarly, FDA, Center for Devices and Radiological Health, Digital Health Center of Excellence is issuing guidance documents related to technologies in clinical research that are supportive of DCTs [6].

One helpful guidance in particular was the "Conduct of Clinical Trials of Medical Products During the COVID-19 Public Health Emergency", draft released in March 2020 and finalized in August 2021. For safety assessments, FDA suggested the implementation of phone contact, virtual visit, or alternative location for assessment, including local labs or imaging centers. Some trial assessments could be delayed, if appropriate; if the assessment could not be properly conducted under the existing protocol, FDA suggested the sponsor to stop ongoing recruitment or even withdraw trial participants. For missing data due to missed visits, changes in trial visits, or participant discontinuations, FDA clarified that sponsors should capture specific information in the case report form that explains the basis of the missing data, including the relationship to COVID-19, for missing protocol-specified information [7]. For investigational products that are typically administered in a health care setting, FDA suggested the use of alternative administration, such as home nursing or alternative sites by trained but non-study personnel. Sponsors were encouraged to consider central and remote monitoring programs for site oversight, as well as consider modifications to the Statistical Analysis Plan on how protocol deviations would be handled. These languages would be similar to the FDA DCT Draft Guidance that would be issued in May 2023.

In the "Digital Health Technologies for Remote Data Acquisition in Clinical Investigations" draft guidance in December 2021, this provided researchers with recommendations on the use of DHTs to acquire data remotely from participants in clinical investigations evaluating medical products. Topics covered are the selection of DHTs for a clinical investigation, verification and validation of DHTs for use in a clinical investigation, use of DHT's measurements as trial endpoints, risks associated with DHTs in a clinical study, and how to manage those risks [8]. Data from DHT measurements allows for more continuous or intermittent recording of physiological, functional and psychological/emotional/behavioral data that may translate to clinical events or characteristics. The ability to transmit data remotely also increases the opportunity for participants to engage in trials at locations remote from the investigator's site. This guidance helped equip trial sponsors with more clarity around the definition of DHTs and tie value with DCT implementation.

Release of the FDA DCT Draft Guidance and Beyond

On May 2, 2023, the FDA released its much-anticipated DCT draft guidance [9]. This guidance defined DCTs and listed out core elements. It also opened new questions for industry researchers. FDA Commissioner Robert Califf believe it is "a major step forward" in the agency's efforts to create "a more robust clinical trial ecosystem." Through this draft guidance, the agency also encourages the use of innovative trial design and health care technologies to advance meaningful evidence generation in clinical trials. Early sentiment from some industry leaders at the 13th annual Disruptive Innovations to Modernize Clinical Research (DPHARM) conference in September 2023 expressed a desire to move away from the term DCTs towards "DCT elements" or "flexible approaches" for clinical trials. Regardless of the terminology wished to be used by the industry, the FDA DCT draft guidance implemented the official regulatory terminology for the field and represents a cohesive step forward for the industry to align on the definitions, priorities, and implementation of DCT strategies and approaches.

As the Guidance is still draft, only specific sections will be highlighted.

Reaffirming the Definition and Value of DCT

FDA defined a DCT as a trial in which some (hybrid DCTs) or all (full DCTs) of the clinical trial-related activities occur away at a clinical trial site which is headed by an investigator, such as a participant's home. The value of DCTs is the opportunity to enhance diversity, improve participant experience, reduce caregiver burden, and facilitate research on rare disease populations and populations with limited mobility. For sponsors, this presents as an opportunity to enhance equity, diversity, and inclusion in trial populations. Using outreach strategies such as local health care institutions (pharmacies, clinics) that may have ties to the community presents as an underutilized resource in the health system to optimize the conduct of clinical research. Bringing DCTs to the places where participants live may also reduce the need for participants to travel to sites and improve participant engagement, recruitment, and retention with challenges accessing traditional sites. Lastly, the use of local healthcare providers (HCPs) may reduce cultural and linguistic barriers to participation in DCTs.

There are also DCT elements already existing in many trials, and the FDA calls out local clinical laboratory facilities, telehealth, and DHTs. Full DCTs may be better suited for trials that do not have complex medical assessments and those with IMPs that have a well-characterized safety profile and are easy to administer. In this guidance, the FDA highlights that the operational complexity to implement a DCT may be high. FDA recommends that a facilitation (communications) plan be put in place that describes the coordination of the planned DCT elements, such as the use of local HCP facilities, local clinical laboratories, visits to participants' homes, direct distribution of investigational products to participants at their locations. Early engagement with FDA review divisions is key to assess for feasibility, design, implementation, and analysis. Notably, the components that are not listed are elements that had historically been pitched to sponsors are: digital payment, eCOA, and tools for increasing participant engagement such as gamification, reminders, and other approaches.

DCT Design

DCTs involve a network of locations, all under investigator oversight, that include trial personnel and non-trial personnel. The trial personnel is not a new concept. The inclusion of non-trial personnel is a newer concept in which local HCPs can perform assessments that are within their medical licensure and that do not require knowledge of the protocol of the investigator's brochure.

The variability and precision of data obtained in a DCT may differ from a traditional site-based trial. FDA provides a well-established example, which is in participant self-administered tests such as home spirometry. The assessments performed by local HCPs as part of routine clinical practice may be more variable and less precise than assessments conducted by trial personnel (e.g.: evaluation of symptoms) and thus, the research team should consider the different statistical analysis to be performed.

The audit trail of a DCT is a similar approach to that of a traditional brick and mortar trial. Therefore, for inspection purposes, there should be a physical location where all clinical trial-related records for participants under the investigator's care are accessible and where trial personnel can be interviewed. Overall, the regulatory requirements and expectations for DCTs are the same as for any other trial.

Remote Visits: Telehealth and Non-trial Personnel

FDA encourages investigators to consider telehealth visits if no in-person interaction is needed and the protocol should specify which visits are appropriate for telehealth visits and when the participant should be seen in-person.

For non-trial personnel, FDA refers to the use of local HCPs for in-person visits that do not require protocol or IMP-specific knowledge. These can be doctors or nurses that are selected to perform activities that do not differ from those that they are qualified to perform in routine clinical practice. Notably, the burden of responsibility falls on the investigators to ensure that the local HCPs are qualified, that the outputs coming in from local HCPs are supervised and adequate (e.g.: data quality). For documentation purposes, there is the introduction of a "Task Log", which is different from the Delegation Log. The Delegation of Authority Log, in which industry shortens to "Delegation Log", is to record all trial staff members that contribute to trial-related activities. Its purpose is to track all individuals who have been trained by the investigator and authorized to perform trial-related tasks and procedures. On the other hand, the Task Log seems to be a separate log that is for local HCPs contracted to provide trial-related services that are part of routine clinical practice. Individuals on the Delegation Log are listed on the Statement of the Investigator, Form FDA 1572. On the other hand, individuals on the Task Log should not be included on the Form FDA 1572.

Responsibilities of the Investigator

The key differences between investigators that run a brick and mortar trial versus investigators that run a DCT with remote elements are the extent to which the investigator uses technology, DHTs, and trial personnel to interact remotely with participants. DCT investigators have the same regulatory responsibility for the conduct of the DCT and oversight of individuals delegated to perform trial-related activities as the investigators of traditional clinical trials. To ensure consistent implementation, customized training, coordination, and SOPs may be required, such as: delegation of trial-related activities to local HCPs, videoconferencing can be used to oversee trial personnel performing activities (e.g., photographing lesions, fitting sensors), and a limit to the number of participants an investigator can appropriately manage. Quality control measures should be in place to reduce data variability, including regular review by investigators to assess for consistency and completeness of the required procedure. Investigators must maintain the task log with all local HCPs that list the name and affiliations, description of roles and assigned tasks, dates these local HCPs were added to the task log, and location of activities to be conducted by local HCPs.

Considerations for Investigational Product

Investigational medical product (IMP) should be administered by investigators or sub-investigators. The nature of IMP is important to determine if appropriate to administer outside of a trial site in a DCT. IMP that may not be appropriate are those with high-risk safety profiles or that the safety profile is not yet well-defined. If the IMP has other safety risks such as hypersensitivity or abuse potential, it may not be appropriate in a DCT.

IMPs that may be appropriate are those with a well-characterized safety profile and that do not require specialized monitoring in the immediate post-administrative setting. Characteristics of IMP that are best suited for direct-to-participant shipment are those with long shelf lives and good stability profiles.

A hybrid DCT can be used for IMPs that require supervised but infrequent administration where the administration is done at a trial site (in-person) but the follow-up is done at a more convenient location (remotely).

Looking Beyond

Many international organizations have convened to discuss and evaluate the principles that govern clinical research and the impact of evolving technologies to existing frameworks. For example, Good Clinical Practice (GCP) is an international ethical and scientific quality standard for designing, conducting, recording, and reporting human clinical trials. The International Council for Harmonisation of Technical Requirements for Pharmaceuticals for Human Use (ICH) was founded in 1990 to bring together regulatory authorities and industry and develop and maintain guidelines for clinical research. As discussed previously in Chap. 2, in May 2023, the ICH E6(R3) Guideline was released that contained principles intended to support efficient approaches to trial design and conduct, citing innovative digital health technologies [10]. ICH E6(R3) supports the use of technologies to be incorporated into existing healthcare infrastructures and enable the use of a variety of relevant data sources in clinical trials. The use of technologies may also encourage wider participation in clinical trials. In addition, the guideline encouraged the involvement of participants in the design of the trial to achieve quality and meaningful trial outcomes. This input will also guide decisions on the feasibility of data collection and assure that participation in the trial does not become unduly burdensome for those involved.

Quiz Questions
1. Which of the following are examples of efforts made by the U.S. government prior to the COVID-19 pandemic to modernize the conduct and regulation of clinical trials?
   (A) Twenty-First Century Cures Act
   (B) FDA Technology Modernization Action Plan
   (C) International Council of Harmonization
   (D) A and B
   (E) B and C
2. Which of the following is INCORRECT regarding the FDA Guidance "Conduct of Clinical Trials of Medical Products During the COVID-19 Public Health Emergency"?
   (A) Modifications to the trial conduct can include using alternative sites by trained non-study personnel
   (B) It did not include information on how to address missing data
   (C) Depending on the nature of the protocol, it may be necessary for sponsors to stop ongoing recruitment or even withdraw trial participants
3. Which of the following is CORRECT regarding the FDA Draft DCT Guidance, released in May 2023?
   (A) Individuals on the Task Log should be added to the Form FDA 1572
   (B) Investigators' scope of responsibility decreases due to the remote nature of trial assessments
   (C) Investigational product in DCTs should have complex medical assessments
   (D) The variability and precision of data obtained in a DCT may differ from a traditional site-based trial

Answers to Quiz Questions
1. D
2. B
3. D

The regulatory landscape continues to evolve rapidly. Pre-competitive industry working groups continue to band together to define and encourage adoption and tracking of DCT elements. One thing is certain: the COVID-19 pandemic accelerated the adoption of DCTs out of necessity and health authorities continue to collaborate closely with industry to better elucidate uncertainty.

Bibliography

1. United States: National Archives and Records Administration: Office of the Federal Register. An act making consolidated appropriations for the fiscal year ending September 30, 2022, and for providing emergency assistance for the situation in Ukraine, and for other purposes. 2022. https://www.govinfo.gov/app/details/PLAW-117publ103. Accessed 10 Dec 2023.
2. Rep. Eshoo AG [D C 18. H.R.7667—117th Congress (2021–2022): Food and Drug Amendments of 2022. 2022. https://www.congress.gov/bill/117th-congress/house-bill/7667. Accessed 10 Dec 2023.
3. World Health Organization (WHO). https://www.who.int. Accessed 10 Dec 2023.
4. Suman A, van Es J, Gardarsdottir H, et al. A cross-sectional survey on the early impact of COVID-19 on the uptake of decentralised trial methods in the conduct of clinical trials. Trials. 2022;23(1):856. https://doi.org/10.1186/s13063-022-06706-x.
5. Health C for D and R. Digital Health Center of Excellence. FDA. 2023. https://www.fda.gov/medical-devices/digital-health-center-excellence. Accessed 10 Dec 2023.
6. Health C for D and R. Guidances with Digital Health Content. FDA. 2023. https://www.fda.gov/medical-devices/digital-health-center-excellence/guidances-digital-health-content. Accessed 10 Dec 2023.
7. Research C for DE and FDA Guidance on Conduct of Clinical Trials of Medical Products During the COVID-19 Public Health Emergency. 2023.

https://www.fda.gov/regulatory-information/search-fda-guidance-documents/fda-guidance-conduct-clinical-trials-medical-products-during-covid-19-public-health-emergency. Accessed 10 Dec 2023.
8. Research C for DE and Digital Health Technologies for Remote Data Acquisition in Clinical Investigations. 2023. https://www.fda.gov/regulatory-information/search-fda-guidance-documents/digital-health-technologies-remote-data-acquisition-clinical-investigations. Accessed 10 Dec 2023.
9. Research C for DE and Decentralized Clinical Trials for Drugs, Biological Products, and Devices. 2023. https://www.fda.gov/regulatory-information/search-fda-guidance-documents/decentralized-clinical-trials-drugs-biological-products-and-devices. Accessed 9 Dec 2023.
10. ICH_E6(R3)_DraftGuideline_2023_0519.pdf. https://database.ich.org/sites/default/files/ICH_E6%28R3%29_DraftGuideline_2023_0519.pdf. Accessed 9 Dec 2023.

Methodology and Protocol Development

Anna H. Yang and Isaac R. Rodriguez-Chavez

Objectives
By the end of this chapter, you will be able to:

1. List and define the roles and responsibilities of the clinical trial team members
2. Briefly describe Trancelerate's existing resources and tools for designing DCTs
3. Explain the impact of decentralized elements to trial protocol design
4. Provide recommendations to Ethics Committee/Institutional Review Board when reviewing DCTs

---

A. H. Yang (✉)
Genentech, A Member of the Roche Group,
South San Francisco, CA, USA

I. R. Rodriguez-Chavez
CEO & Principal Independent Consultant, Scientific, Clinical, Regulatory Affairs and Digital Health Technologies, 4Biosolutions Consulting, Rockville, MD, USA

© The Author(s), under exclusive license to Springer Nature Switzerland AG 2024
A. H. Yang, I. R. Rodriguez-Chavez (eds.), *Fundamentals of Decentralized Clinical Trials*,
https://doi.org/10.1007/978-3-031-62877-1_4

Introduction to the Clinical Trial Team

A flexible approach using decentralized methodology should be the default consideration when planning a new trial. Prior to finalizing the DCT protocol, the discussion of remote procedures and flexible participation should be assessed to ensure logistical feasibility. Depending on the team's resource allocation such as timelines, budget, and the clinical development plan of the molecule to be studied in the trial, certain restrictions are in place. The team should determine the prioritized areas of evidence generation, such as more participant-generated data (e.g., eCOA, biosensors), the opportunity to enroll broader participants (e.g., non-ambulatory, rural, ethnicity, etc), remote assessments (e.g., mobile phlebotomy, remote scans, remote physical assessments), direct-to-participant shipment, virtual investigator or trial team, or utilizing telehealth to facilitate virtual conversations and check-ins. In this chapter, we will discuss key sections of a clinical trial protocol and provide insight into what modifications should be considered.

Clinical Research Team

Though varied by institution, a typical clinical research team usually comprises of some or all the following members:

- Primary Investigator of a grant, cooperative agreement, or contract: primary individual responsible for the preparation, conduct, and administration of a research grant, cooperative agreement, training or public service project, contract, or other sponsored project in compliance with applicable laws and regulations and institutional policy governing the conduct of sponsored research
- Investigator of a clinical investigation: is the individual who actually conducts a clinical investigation (i.e., under whose immediate direction the test article is administered or dis-

pensed to, or used involving, a subject) or, in the event of an investigation conducted by a team of individuals, is the responsible leader of that team [1].
- Sub-Investigator: key personnel also responsible for the conduct of the trial. The investigator is the ultimate person responsible, but SI is also obligated to ensure the project is conducted in compliance with applicable laws and regulations and institutional policy governing the conduct of sponsored research.
- Co-Investigator (Co-I) of a grant, cooperative agreement, or contract: One of two individuals designated by the applicant organization to have the appropriate level of authority and responsibility to direct the project or program to be supported by the award.
- Clinical Research Coordinator or Manager: supervises the program, maintains quality assurance, coordinates with Investigator and/or SI to ensure that the clinical trial investigator responsibilities are met, manages site staffing, oversees the budget, prepares for audits, ensure appropriate delegation of responsibilities among research team.
- Clinical Research Associate: screening potential participants, preparing documents and slides for institutional review board and ethics committee submission, filing protocol amendments, coordinating participant calendars.
- Research nurses: screening potential participants, determining eligibility, submitting safety data, conducting participant education, assessing potential adverse events.
- Research pharmacists: screening potential participants, determining eligibility, conducting participant education, assessing potential adverse events.

Depending on the technology partner utilized, the following additional resources may be added to the team:

- Digital Navigator: An individual trained to support participants and site staff with technology-related issues that affect the understanding and conduct of the trial.

- Virtual research coordinator: An individual that may not be employed by the site to support with delegation of clinical research associate or clinical research coordinator tasks.
- Home Health Nurses: Medically trained professionals employed by the site or by vendors that are trained to administer IMPs and assess/collect information for the clinical trial.
- Service support: Individuals available to participants and site for 24/7 hotline support on technology-related issues.

Impact of Decentralized Elements to the Trial Team

How Might a DCT Affect the Team?

When designing a study with DCT elements, study teams should survey the end user to ensure feasibility. Scientific rigor is important but operational feasibility and ease of execution is important to get right so the trial is completed effectively. Are these endpoints typically collected as part of clinical practice? Are these endpoints collected at their institution? By which instruments or DHTs? Survey the participants; give an estimate of how long the activities would take. Would participating in these activities be a burden? Could you foresee yourself staying in the trial for the [x] months required? Would you rather come in less frequently for longer visits each time, or more frequently for a shorter time? After surveying the participants and sites, it's time to write the flexibility into the protocol.

Of note, the Modernizing Clinical Trial Conduct (MCTC) initiative established within the nonprofit organization, Transcelerate, developed several publicly available resources for clinical research teams to use as they implement DCT elements in their protocol [2]. These resources are a combination of data and qualitative experience from industry learnings around the successes and challenges of technology services. One resource is the Operational Complexity Assessment Tool (OCAT), which is an exercise for trial teams to think through the operational complexities of components of their trial protocol. Based on the level of operational complexity, this tool helps trial teams organize potential supportive measures to mitigate the complexity. The different categories for consideration are digital data, direct to participant shipment, eConsent, home health visits, local facilities, remote site monitoring, and telemedicine.

MCTC also released several Process Frameworks in 2021 associated with each category. These Frameworks provide detailed explanations of considerations at each stage of the trial planning and implementation process. These considerations align with traditional considerations during a brick and mortar trial set-up, for example: evaluating and defining timelines for contracting vendors and site logistics during the trial start-up phase. Novel considerations are also provided, for example: Considering how the digital data will be stored for future use in the development of new algorithms during the trial closeout and reporting phase.

During the COVID-19 pandemic, there was a surge of interest and dedication from the industry to come together and gather learnings and create resources for future trial teams. The MCTC initiative is one such example. In the immediate months following the COVID-19 pandemic, early signs from the pharmaceutical industry indicate that perhaps a separate team with dedicated expertise is needed to provide guidance or implementation strategies for trial teams. There remains a challenge to train up teams in this space, given the magnitude of fragmented information.

How to Write a Flexible Protocol for Decentralized Elements

In this portion, we will use a hypothetical full DCT to discuss how the strategy and execution of the trial was described in the protocol. Note that every trial and every Sponsor is different. The goal of this section is to put into action the strategy of DCTs into execution.

- Trial Title: Proof-of-concept of a full DCT in a large integrated health delivery network using telehealth, a DHT for remote

monitoring, local facilities, and direct-to-participant shipment (n = 80)
- Participant population: Participants with advanced cancer, Eastern Cooperative Oncology Group (ECOG) performance status = 0–2
- Intervention: Standard-of-care treatment

Trial Objectives and Trial Endpoints

The objective of this trial is to prove feasibility of a DCT model. To date, the overall industry comfort level is to limit DCTs in non-label-enabling studies, such as phase IV post-marketing long-term follow-up studies. Some companies have also converted Expanded Access Program (EAP) studies into hybrid DCTs to provide even greater flexible pathways for participants with serious or immediately life-threatening disease or condition to gain access to an investigational medical product outside a clinical trial. There are also some companies, such as Boehringer Ingelheim, that have implemented a full DCT as a mirror design to a label-enabling phase II clinical trial with a New Molecular Entity (NME) for treatment of major depressive disorder. Eventually, the industry will move to apply DCT more to label-enabling phase III and earlier studies.

In this trial, feasibility is the trial objective. Feasibility to demonstrate the DCT model can help to establish baseline comfort in a remote approach to clinical trials. Participants will be receiving their standard-of-care treatment with the DCT model as the intervention of providing flexible clinical care. The independent variable is the set-up of the DCT model, and the dependent variables can be participant satisfaction, participant adoption, geographic reach of participants, and participant retention.

These dependent variables can then be grouped as the definition of feasibility. The most meaningful dependent variable should be selected as the calculation for sample size.

- Participant satisfaction
- Participant adoption of telehealth or other technology services

- Ability to reach a broader participant population
- *Participant retention → this can be selected as the most meaningful, and therefore, the calculation of sample size and the statistical analysis plan can be centered around this endpoint. Depending on the duration of the trial, select a meaningful time point. Example: for a 1-year feasibility trial, participant retention can be measured at 6 months.*

Trial Design

Through conversations with the Investigator, the trial team should define a chain of communication and participant handoffs. The language in the final protocol should be clear but not too limiting. Define clearly what the responsibilities are for the Investigator, for example: pre-screening participants, diagnosis, treatment, and management of participants, data review, and data entry. The flow of participant onboarding should also be described here, including the training for using the digital health technologies (DHTs) and using the telehealth platform.

1. Complete eConsent
2. Train the participant on the DHT and telehealth platform
3. Investigator to provide individual treatment recommendations
4. Follow up for 6 months using telehealth and measure ongoing satisfaction
5. At 6 months, complete exit questionnaire

There is also a concept of building the "site" around the participant for flexibility, as described by the Society for Clinical Research Sites [3]. Consider listing out all the different remote components that different participants may need and experience. For example:

- Participant A lives very close to the clinic and does not need flexibility—clinic only
- Participant B lives 1 h away from the clinic but 20 min away from their local HCP—local HCP, clinic, telehealth

- Participant C lives 2 h away from the clinic and 1 h away from their local HCP; cannot attend most in-person visits—eConsent, mobile health, DtP, telehealth

Since this is a feasibility trial, certain components are mandatory, such as eConsent, telehealth, and the DHT.

In other studies that are currently deploying DCT elements in a hybrid approach, a common theme is arising—every component should be provided as an option, but never be made mandatory.

Inclusion and Exclusion Criteria

This should not be modified to serve the DCT model. Keep the clinical disease-specific inclusion and exclusion criteria. Since this is a full DCT, participants may experience systemic technology barriers: Not having access to a landline or WiFi connection. It is important *not* to exclude these participants.

Data Sources

This trial contains non-electronic case report forms (eCRF) and eCRF data sources. Here, the trial team can list out all the sources of data. This includes telehealth platform, electronic medical record, DHT data, and any datasets to track participant diversity. To account for the several sources of data, the FDA Draft Guidance recommends trial teams to implement a Data Management Plan (DMP). Implemented into a trial protocol, this can look like:

- Data collected during the enrollment period: disease-specific data
- Data collected during the observation period: DHT information, disease-specific data, satisfaction
- Data collected at trial completion: DHT information, disease-specific data, satisfaction

- Data quality assurance: Update the standard language with any methods used for remote data acquisition from trial participants, trial personnel, and contracted service providers

FDA recommends that the DMP contain a diagram that follows the flow of data from origin to final storage. Due to the potential shifting nature of vendors and technologies used in studies, the protocol should list the *type* of technology used, not the vendor name: example: telehealth platform instead of "Zoom" or "FaceTime".

Preparations Considerations for Ethics Committees and Investigational Review Boards

Ethics Committees (ECs) may challenge the justification of using a DCT approach over site-based traditional trials. While ECs do recognize the potential added value of DCTs, they may anticipate DCTs to be more burdensome and less safe. In order to capture this perspective, a case trial of three EC groups reviewed a DCT protocol that investigated the real-world use of long-acting insulin versus basal insulin through a multinational, phase IV, randomized, open-label approach [4]. The EC members in this trial expressed predominantly hesitant attitudes and questioned the validity and accuracy of data, fair participant selection due to the level of digital literacy required, and maintenance of participant safety due to fewer in-person visits. The authors who critiqued this trial hypothesize that the EC hesitancy may be due to the historical context of regulatory oversight in clinical research. Regulators consider research to be inherently risky for participants and adding novel concepts such as DCTs, especially with the industry's current limited experience and evidence, may bring more uncertainty.

Therefore, when presenting a DCT to EC, trial teams should present the concept as a sliding scale, not an all-or-nothing approach. Each DCT element should be justified. The burden to participants should be weighed in terms of time and resources, and clearly described in the informed consents.

Similarly, Investigational Reviews Boards (IRB) recognize the ethical and regulatory challenges of emerging technologies, not limited to DCTs, and have outlined the need for shared and dynamic resources that improve awareness and understanding of technologies to maintain participant privacy and data confidentiality [5].

Multi-Regional Clinical Trials and Medable Task Force for IRB/EC Considerations for DCT Review

In June 2023, the Multi-Regional Clinical Trials (MRCT) Leadership Task Force released a guidance document around IRB/EC considerations. In order to maintain quality, privacy, and security, please review the select recommendations made to IRB/EC. A complete list of recommendations can be found above in Nebeker et al.'s publication in 2017.

- People
  - Recruitment: Provide a list of online recruitment methods, including the script of information and images, and whether this is passive or active. Ensure the method is aligned with local laws and regulations.
  - eConsent: Language should be consistent with regular consent. Provide a method for verification of identification for the participant. Ensure the platform is secure and that the storage of eConsent records is reviewed.
  - DtP: Ensure requirements of Good Manufacturing Practice (GMP) and Good Distribution Practice (GDP) are met. Review where the IMP will be shipped, what interstate laws must be adhered to, storage conditions, documentation requirements, and accountability/chain of custody.
  - Participants and Technology: Ensure equitable access to the trial, ensure adequate participant education and training, ensure privacy/confidentiality considerations, and review impact to special populations (e.g., pediatrics, prisoners).

- Notifications and Reminders: Consider undue burden to participants, consider minimization of potentially sensitive and confidential information.
- Help Desk: Ensure that the Help Desk is NOT providing medical advice. Look for a clear separation of scope within the Help Desk for technical versus protocol-specific questions. Calls should be logged for audit purposes; there should be no record linking the identity of the caller to the trial or condition.
- Rewards: The IRB/EC should be provided with a summary of how the incentive system is designed
- Data Collection
  - Telehealth: Consider participant preferences for interacting with the trial team, the nature of the interactions and if another caregiver or clinical team member needs to be present, privacy of the participants, any language translation needed, data privacy and security in collection, storage, and transfer.
  - In-home visits: Ensure the in-home visits are appropriate. Consider time and expenses to the site, regulatory and administrative issues with third-party vendor contracting, challenges to Investigator oversight, ability to provide emergency care, access to specialized equipment, and address concerns for maintaining data security and transfer.
  - Local Providers: Training of local providers must be provided and assured, assurance of Investigator oversight, responsibility grid for providers, data security and privacy for data collection, transfer, and storage
  - Devices (smartphones, tablets): equity and equitable access, minimal set of requirements for BYOD hardware and software should be predefined, ensure PHI and clinical trial data are encrypted at rest and in transit
  - Sensors: Review the intended use and FDA classification of the sensor, determine burden to participants, how the data is stored and transferred, and determine if the sensor will be returned or kept at the end of the trial.

- Data Oversight
  - Trial closeout: Ensure only necessary personal identifying data are retained, review appropriate documentation and closeout activities.
  - Real-time monitoring: Determine type of data available to participants and trial investigators, ensure the site has appropriate resources in place to support DCT requirements of real-time monitoring.

Looking Ahead

Three skill sets are critical for success in innovative work in medicine: a strong clinical background, an even stronger understanding of technology, and an understanding in behavioral change management. Truly understanding the clinical need to pull a health technology solution requires this clinical perspective, but the solution would never be implemented if its duplicates workflow, adds extra clicks to the process, requires additional training, or demands more specialized personnel to support. Change management is critical to influence stakeholders across the industry to recognize the need for change. Dr. Rita McGrath from the Columbia Business School points out that for a transformation to happen, there needs to be (1) dissatisfaction with the current state of affairs (2) a vision for the change and (3) understanding of the processes needed to change.

This chapter provides a deeper understanding of (3), the process of writing a clinical trial and getting the trial approved through the necessary EC and IRB committees. Along with a strong clinical and technology background, new clinical trialists like yourself can create meaningful and lasting change for participants so that clinical trial participation is seen only as an opportunity, not a burden.

Quiz Questions

1. Which of the following is an INACCURATE description of the following clinical research team?
   (A) *Primary Investigator (PI) of a grant, cooperative agreement, or contract*: primary individual responsible for the preparation, conduct, and administration of a research grant, cooperative agreement, training or public service project, contract, or other sponsored project in compliance with applicable laws and regulations and institutional policy governing the conduct of sponsored research
   (B) *Sub-Investigator*: vendor contracted to help prescreen participants, hired by the Sponsor company as an assistant to the pharmacy team
   (C) *Clinical Research Associate*: screening potential participants, preparing documents and slides for institutional review board and ethics committee submission, filing protocol amendments, coordinating participant calendars
   (D) *Research pharmacists*: screening potential participants, determining eligibility, conducting participant education, assessing potential adverse events
2. What is the name of the tool developed by Transcelerate that helps trial teams think through operational complexities of their protocol?
   (A) Institutional Review Board
   (B) Operational Complexities Framework
   (C) Process Framework
   (D) Operational Complexity Assessment Tool
3. Which of the following dependent variables is most meaningful to deploy to measure feasibility of a DCT?
   (A) participant satisfaction
   (B) participant retention
   (C) Safety events
   (D) Efficacy of the IND

4. What are the core values for EC/IRB committees to keep in mind when evaluating DCT studies?
   (A) Quality, privacy, and security
   (B) Confidentiality, scientific rigor, enrolling only digitally literate participants
   (C) Change management, operational complexity, speed to market
   (D) Global impact, sustainability, regulatory policy

Answers to Quiz Questions
1. B
2. D
3. B
4. A

Bibliography

1. eCFR::21 CFR Part 312—Investigational New Drug Application. https://www.ecfr.gov/current/title-21/chapter-I/subchapter-D/part-312. Accessed 10 Dec 2023.
2. Modernizing Clinical Trial Conduct. TransCelerate. https://www.transceleratebiopharmainc.com/initiatives/modernizing-clinical-trial-conduct/. Accessed 10 Dec 2023.
3. Vulcano D. Society for Clinical Research Sites Survey Results 2023. Presented at: Operationalize Decentralized Clinical Trials Summit; September 18, 2023; Philadelphia, PA.
4. Van Rijssel TI, De Jong AJ, Santa-Ana-Tellez Y, Boeckhout M, Zuidgeest MGP, Van Thiel GJMW. Ethics review of decentralized clinical trials (DCTs): results of a mock ethics review. Drug Discov Today. 2022;27(10):103326. https://doi.org/10.1016/j.drudis.2022.07.011.
5. Nebeker C, Harlow J, Espinoza Giacinto R, Orozco-Linares R, Bloss CS, Weibel N. Ethical and regulatory challenges of research using pervasive sensing and other emerging technologies: IRB perspectives. AJOB Empir Bioeth. 2017;8(4):266–76. https://doi.org/10.1080/23294515.2017.1403980.

Goals and Metrics of Success

Isaac R. Rodriguez-Chavez, Anna H. Yang, Jane Myles, and Shelly Barnes

Objectives
By the end of this chapter, you will be able to:

1. List metrics and key performance indicators set by pre-competitive industry groups.
2. Apply these principles and schools of thought to trial designs.
3. Develop an understanding of how to implement metrics to future scalability trials.

I. R. Rodriguez-Chavez
CEO & Principal Independent Consultant, Scientific, Clinical, Regulatory Affairs and Digital Health Technologies, 4Biosolutions Consulting, Rockville, MD, USA

A. H. Yang (✉)
Genentech, A Member of the Roche Group,
South San Francisco, CA, USA

J. Myles
Decentralized Trials and Research Alliance, San Diego, CA, USA
e-mail: jane.myles@dtra.org

S. Barnes
UCB, Brussels, Belgium, USA
e-mail: shelly.barnes@ucb.com

© The Author(s), under exclusive license to Springer Nature Switzerland AG 2024
A. H. Yang, I. R. Rodriguez-Chavez (eds.), *Fundamentals of Decentralized Clinical Trials*,
https://doi.org/10.1007/978-3-031-62877-1_5

Background and Commentary

The value of implementing DCT elements is theoretically positive, and researchers are diligently convening to create a unified methodology to benchmark and track success. As science and medicine advances, the way a clinical trial is conducted matters almost equally. This can be tracked using, for example, participant experience, diversity, and ability to reduce burden of participant and caregiver participation.

This section will discuss non-financial metrics. There is emerging data from the Tufts Center for the Study of Drug Development (CSDD) on the financial savings that DCTs can offer [1]. Tufts CSDD and Medable conducted a study to examine the expected Net Present Value (eNPV) of DCTs. NPV is a financial metric used to assess whether a project is economically viable. The "expected" in eNPV indicates that the calculation incorporates probabilities or likelihoods of different outcomes, as many investments are associated with varying levels of risk and uncertainty. It is commonly employed in the drug development industry. A positive NPV indicates a financially sound investment that is expected to generate more cash inflows than outflows, while a negative NPV suggests that the investment is not likely to be profitable.

Tufts included protocols that were finalized between January 2013 to December 2018 that met any of the following DCT elements: Contained data from devices and apps such as electronic clinical outcome assessments, diaries, and connected sensors, real-world evidence, or electronic health records (EHRs). In their analysis of 160 phase II and phase III protocols, Tufts CSDD found a clear positive financial benefit to deploying DCT elements. For phase II trials, a $two million investment can result in a $ten million return and in phase III trials, a $three million investment can yield a $39 million return. For implementation costs, the study used data from Medable based on average contract values for the period between 2020 and 2021. These findings suggest early signs that DCT approaches could have meaningful financial benefits for pharmaceutical endeavors and are worth considering by industry stakeholders.

These are very early results. Caution should be exercised to not broadly extrapolate these findings. For the current state of a rapidly developing space, it may be more prudent to develop non-financial metrics. Many groups have already published early metrics and there is a growing alignment across industry regarding impact measures for DCT approaches.

Early Metrics of Success

The Decentralized Trials and Research Alliance (DTRA) is a pre-competitive cross-ecosystem collaboration that brings together early adopters of DCTs, including representatives from biopharmaceutical sponsors, technology partners, contract research organizations, research sites and institutions, regulatory bodies, and other leading health technology trailblazers. DTRA and its Leadership Council chartered 12 cross-functional initiative teams, such as "Mapping the Participant Journey", "Data Connectivity", and "Key Performance Indicators". The Key Performance Indicators (KPIs) team, consolidated over 70 metrics to 10 that aim to measure success in both hybrid and full DCTs relative to traditional trials. Each of these 10 metrics will be discussed in depth.

As of 2023, there is no simple way to track either the adoption or impact of DCT approaches. This is in part because these trials are not consistently listed in trial registries such as ClinicalTrials.gov or other federal registries. This means it's not simple to compare the impact of DCT approaches to traditional approaches in similar trials, by therapeutic area, size, phase, or other parameters. Impact may be being measured at an individual organization or even trial team level—but is not readily available to help create best practices for DCT use. Furthermore, the impact measures may not be consistent or comparable from one organization or team to another. The gap in objective data to measure impact has been recognized across the clinical trials ecosystem. As of mid-2023, Tufts Center for the Study of Drug Development is collaborating with several pharmaceutical and biotech organizations to collect initial data to measure DCT impact. By mid-2024 there may be some initial analysis to help quantify both the adoption and initial impact of DCT approaches.

Key Performance Indicators: A Closer Look
1. Likelihood to engage in a DCT
2. Participant drop-out rate due to a participant decision
3. Number of adverse events reported per number of randomized participants
4. Speed, in terms of enrollment rate
5. Diversity and inclusion
6. Cost
7. Participant load per site
8. Database lock timelines
9. Compliance
10. Inclusion of participants in a clinical trial due to DCT facility

Metric 1. Likelihood to Engage in a DCT

In addition to clinical effectiveness and participant safety, participant experience is the third pillar for healthcare quality. A systematic review of 55 trials that included a wide range of demographic groups of various ages concluded that there are positive associations between participant experience and health outcomes. Positive participant experiences were connected with greater adherence to recommended clinical practice and medication, preventative care, and less resource use such as hospitalization and primary care visits [2].

Embedding participant satisfaction surveys before, during, or after the trial are all acceptable ways to capture participant satisfaction. The Transcelerate Study Participant Feedback Questionnaire (SFPQ) [3] provides sample questions for all three time points, and has been recently updated to align to DCT approaches. Some suggested topics to survey participant are the following:

- Prior to the trial: Comfort level, trust, foreseen barriers to participation
- During the trial: Comfort level, trust, ease of participation
- After the trial: Comfort level, trust, unforeseen barriers to participation

As a best practice, these questions should be validated by Sponsor and/or the academic center's participant-reported outcomes (PROs) group.

Site satisfaction or site adoption could also be measured at different points in time. Metrics around how to define this exactly is yet to be determined and agreed upon by the industry.

Metric 2. Participant Dropout Percentage Due to Participant Decision

Participant dropout due to the participant's decision, including participant lost to follow-up, is important to track for purposes of measuring patient retention. This is essentially tracking retention due to voluntary participant choice, not clinical or safety factors. Conflicting opinions exist regarding whether technology can alienate some participants or create the optionality and flexibility for the trial to fit into the lives of participants. In a pivotal survey conducted by the American Cancer Society during the COVID-19 pandemic, the researchers asked, "What is the association of remote technology and other decentralization tools with participant likelihood to enroll in cancer clinical trials?" Of nearly 1200 participants, most respondents (ranging from 60 to 85%) stated they would be more likely to enroll in a cancer clinical trial if remote technology and other tools reduced the need for travel to a trial site [4]. The survey included mostly White (70%) female (75%) respondents receiving treatment or already received treatment for breast cancer (41%). The survey has some limitations; participation intent does not always correlate to actual participation, the questions are not specific to a clinical trial phase, and there may be participation bias, as respondents taking part in survey research may be more predisposed to research in general. This metric, if applied broadly across Sponsors, will prove to be one way to measure the actual retention of participant on a trial.

Metric 3. Number of Adverse Events Reported Per Number of Randomized Participants

The number of adverse events (AEs) and serious adverse events (SAEs) for a DCT should be similar to the AEs and SAEs in a traditional trial. The rationale to quantify safety reporting is that remotely managing participants will not pose more harm to participants compared to if they were to be managed in the traditional manner. Total AE reports is a highly correlated to therapeutic area, disease state, and drug safety profile and we caution against generalized cross-trial AE comparisons. If applicable, the trial team should track the total number of AEs and SAEs reported by remote participants vs traditional participants that are being overseen with brick and mortar approaches.

Depending on the nature of the trial, participants may be able to report AEs at their local HCPs' facility. Trial teams should identify, along with the investigators of the trial, which adverse events must be treated at physical locations and which AEs can be handled via telehealth. Some participants may require an in-person assessment or additional diagnostic tests for further evaluation, which should also be clearly documented in the protocol.

Metric 4. Speed Through Enrollment Rate

There is a standing hypothesis that the duration between First Patient In (FPI) and Last Patient In (LPI) is shorter using decentralized recruitment approaches. Another possible comparative metric is the enrollment rate per month per site. This may also be highly therapeutic area, disease, and drug dependent. If the trial involves both brick and mortar and DCT sites, the speed of enrollment may be directly compared. As with all trials, it's highly recommended to understand which recruitment tactics are effective in both virtual and traditional sites, and to compare for similarities and differences (e.g., social media vs EHR recruitment and enrollment success).

Metric 5. Diversity and Inclusion

There is great hope that DCT approaches can play a pivotal role in enabling participant diversity and support inclusion of underserved participant populations. While the importance of tracking race/ethnicity is widely recognized, it is equally imperative for sponsors to consider other key factors such as age, sex, geography, and cultural/heritage needs. There is directional evidence that DCT approaches can help support diverse participation, when combined with trusted, in-community awareness events and recruitment tactics.

Diversity in geography relates to enrolling individuals that reside in rural, remote, metropolitan, and suburban areas. Different geographies may face different barriers to clinical trial participation. For example, participants in metropolitan areas may not own a motorized vehicle due to the nature/cost of urban living. The clinical trial site may not be in a metropolitan area and these participants are therefore unable to travel to the site easily. Patients in rural areas may have motorized vehicles with nearby access to routine care but have no nearby clinical trial sites. DCT elements can broaden the geographic reach for researchers and unlock clinical trial participation for all geographies. By leveraging remote technologies in DCTs, researchers can now enroll participants located hundreds of miles away, thereby breaking down geographical barriers and fostering greater diversity and inclusion in trial populations. As trial teams plan to measure geographic diversity, it will be critical to establish how to assess the participant's geographic location relative to the site, while maintaining appropriate privacy requirements. This geographic location of the participant may need to be tracked by a third-party vendor rather than the trial sponsor to maintain privacy and the Health Insurance Portability and Accountability Act (HIPAA) requirements.

One example on how industry leaders are measuring and trying to improve diversity is related to participant access. For example, Walgreens has three internal metrics to determine success in its clinical trial business: Access, participant comprehension, and pharmacist and clinician training. Since communities of color oftentimes have limited broadband access, Walgreens is working with organizations like Verizon to leverage federal programs and remove systemic barriers so that patients are able to enroll—and stay enrolled in—clinical trials [5]. Most DCT-enabled trials will require participant access to internet services, so systematic approaches to supporting access to broadband critically important to successful operationalization/trial conduct.

Metric 6. Cost

The key cost drivers of pharmaceutical trials in the U.S. across all trial phases are clinical procedure costs (15–22% of total), administrative staff costs (11–29% of total), and site monitoring costs (9–14% of total) [6]. The initial implementation costs of DCT approaches may be higher, until the efficiency of scale across multiple trials and platforms is achieved. Earlier in this chapter, the emerging research from Tufts on the potential financial return of DCTs was discussed. The purpose of this metric is to track the planned versus actual spend on implementing DCT elements. Measuring benefit to the business is not the intention of this metric.

It is essential to consider both the total trial budget (planned and actual) and the specific costs of DCT elements (e.g., technology platforms, DHTs, home nursing). By closely monitoring these costs, researchers can make informed budgetary decisions for efficient trial management. Measuring these costs can also create visibility on up-front costs (e.g. platform development) versus service-based costs (e.g. in-home trial visit costs). These financial elements will be helpful to teams and business units as they plan future trial budgets and can better understand the timing and magnitude of different cost elements.

Metric 7. Participant Load Per Site

Participant load per site is a critical metric to assess DCT impact. DCTs offer potential benefits of expanded reach and leveraging local HCPs, allowing sites to handle more participants efficiently. The use of local HCPs is a new concept in clinical research and its adoption may take some time. This metric evaluates how DCT elements enable sites to enroll and effectively oversee larger numbers of participants s compared to traditional brick-and-mortar sites. Assessing participant load per site in DCTs provides valuable insights into optimizing site workload, enhancing participant recruitment and optimizing participant oversight in trials.

Metric 8. Database Lock Timelines

Trial teams will face the challenge of managing multiple databases and systems, leading to concerns about potential impacts on trial timelines. Vendors may claim that their systems offer seamless integration, but it is essential to critically evaluate such assertions. The level of integration and its actual impact on data analysis need thorough examination to ensure efficient and accurate trial outcomes. Striking the right balance between system complexity and seamless integration is crucial for optimizing study management and data analysis processes.

Metric 9. Compliance

Using DCT approaches may increase complexity and/or introduce new processes to trials. Decreased compliance may be a risk and therefore should be measured. Data collection complexity may also increase, due to increased data volume (number of data points), increased data sources (number of data platforms) or increase data entry points (e.g. site staff, trial services staff, and or participants). This heightened intricacy may increase site protocol deviations. Additionally, the introduction of alerts and reminders may enhance participant compliance to trial assessment completion and data reporting. Assessing the effectiveness of such measures in improving participant compliance is essential for ensuring the successful execution of the trial and accurate data collection.

Metric 10. Inclusion of Participants in a Clinical Trial Due to DCT Facility

This metric is designed to capture participants who were willing but not able to participate in a clinical trial due to barriers traveling to the brick-and-mortar site. Due to the DCT nature—through technology and operational flexibility—the participants can be rescreened and included in the trial.

The CATORI trial, conducted by Genentech, was the first hybrid decentralized clinical trial to utilize the DTRA KPIs to benchmark and begin to measure success of a DCT. An analog of Metric 10 was used during this initial use case: Measuring which participants the brick and mortar site required repeated support such as rideshare, reimbursement, and digital navigator support. The non-interventional study also tracked how many sites needed virtual research coordinator support as part of resource management.

Applying These Metrics to Trial Design

What makes a good clinical trial? According to a draft guidance by the World Health Organization (WHO) for Best Practices for Clinical Trials, "good trials" are reliably informative, ethical, and efficient and answer scientifically important questions relevant to the population they are intended to study, with findings generalizable to those populations. It is widely known that randomized controlled trials (RCTs) are conducted under carefully curated, idealized, and rigorously controlled conditions that may compromise their external validity [7]. Randomized controlled trials demonstrate efficacy of a new therapeutic but not effectiveness. Decentralized clinical trials, given their inclusive nature and flexible data collection outside the site setting, may offer a different framework to of conduct research that is be more representative of the real-world setting and therefore bridge the "efficacy-effectiveness" gap [8].

Careful consideration of which key performance indicators matter most to a specific protocol will help the trial team set up their trial design and choose the appropriate study configuration. It's important to define and align on the key problems to be solved to successfully design and implement a trial, and the KPIs selected need to support the key measures of operational success for the trial. Note that these metrics are not assessing the clinical outcomes of the trial, but rather are focused on measuring if the clinical trial methods being used support the successful conduct of the trial and are "best-fit" for the most important challenges of the trial.

Using multiple vendors increases the number of variables and the risk of the data collection process. Try to use as few vendors as possible and leverage existing services or technology that sites are comfortable with or already using. For example, when mobile nursing is a consideration, work with the sites to determine if using their in-house mobile nurses are an option. Then, write this into the protocol that sites may be able to leverage existing local HCPs already contracted in their healthcare system. Whether using one vendor or many, it's important to understand which operational data points will be needed to measure the agreed-upon KPIs, and to map where the data will come from. Establish the metrics plan as early in the clinical trial planning process as possible to ensure clear expectations are set on what will be measured, who will contribute the data, and how the measures will be calculated.

Closing

These metrics are just a first start in a rapidly evolving space. DCTs—and specifically tracking success and defining value—are still being discussed across the clinical trial ecosystem. There is a strong interest in measuring and quantifying both financial and non-financial impact of DCT approaches, and this data gathering is in early stages as of 2023. As students and future clinical trialists in this exciting space, you are now prepared to synthesize your own takeaways and approach the stage with insightful debate.

> **Quiz Questions**
> 1. Which of the following is INCORRECT in describing the Tufts CSDD's eNPV research on ROI in DCTs?
>   (A) The researchers examined phase I–III trials
>   (B) For phase 2 trials, a $2 million investment can result in a $10 million return
>   (C) The average implementation cost for a phase III DCT trial is $1,042,000 compared to $3,126,000 for traditional phase III trial
>   (D) Tufts CSDD worked with a technology platform vendor to curate the data
> 2. Which of the following is TRUE about the DTRA KPIs effort?
>   (I) Over 70 metrics were collected and consolidated into 10 metrics
>   (II) The team comprised of strictly academic investigators
>   (III) Re-inclusion of participants on a trial due to DCT facility is a key business metric
>   (A) I only
>   (B) I and II only
>   (C) II and III only
>   (D) I and III only
> 3. When speaking with a site, you hear: "If I participate in DCTs, I will lose money". Which metric is most helpful to help you make a case that workload can be optimized through increased productivity of participants management?
>   (A) Database lock timelines
>   (B) Participant load per site
>   (C) Number of adverse events reported
>   (D) Diversity and inclusion

Answers to Quiz Questions
1. A
2. D
3. B

Bibliography

1. DiMasi JA, Smith Z, Oakley-Girvan I, et al. Assessing the financial value of decentralized clinical trials. Ther Innov Regul Sci. 2023;57(2):209–19. https://doi.org/10.1007/s43441-022-00454-5.
2. Doyle C, Lennox L, Bell D. A systematic review of evidence on the links between patient experience and clinical safety and effectiveness. BMJ Open. 2013;3(1):e001570. https://doi.org/10.1136/bmjopen-2012-001570.
3. Study Participant Feedback Questionnaire Toolkit—TransCelerate. https://www.transceleratebiopharmainc.com/assets/patientexperience/study-participant-feedback-questionnaire/. Accessed 9 Dec 2023.
4. Adams DV, Long S, Fleury ME. Association of remote technology use and other decentralization tools with patient likelihood to enroll in cancer clinical trials. JAMA Netw Open. 2022;5(7):e2220053. https://doi.org/10.1001/jamanetworkopen.2022.20053.
5. How Walgreens recruits patients of color for clinical trials. https://www.healthcare-brew.com/stories/2023/07/10/how-walgreens-recruits-patients-of-color-for-clinical-trials. Accessed 9 Dec 2023.
6. Sertkaya A, Wong HH, Jessup A, Beleche T. Key cost drivers of pharmaceutical clinical trials in the United States. Clin Trials. 2016;13(2):117–26. https://doi.org/10.1177/1740774515625964.
7. Fogel DB. Factors associated with clinical trials that fail and opportunities for improving the likelihood of success: a review. Contemp Clin Trials Commun. 2018;11:156–64. https://doi.org/10.1016/j.conctc.2018.08.001.
8. De Brouwer W, Patel CJ, Manrai AK, Rodriguez-Chavez IR, Shah NR. Empowering clinical research in a decentralized world. Npj Digit Med. 2021;4(1):102. https://doi.org/10.1038/s41746-021-00473-w.

Correction to: Fundamentals of Decentralized Clinical Trials

Anna H. Yang
and Isaac R. Rodriguez-Chavez

Correction to:
A. H. Yang, I. R. Rodriguez-Chavez (Eds.),
Fundamentals of Decentralized Clinical Trials,
https://doi.org/10.1007/978-3-031-62877-1

This book was inadvertently published with incorrect affiliation for the author "Craig Lipset" in the Foreword and authors "Anna H. Yang and Isaac R. Rodriguez-Chavez" in the Front Matter and Chapters 2, 3, 4, and 5.

Front Matter

The affiliation for the editor Isaac R. Rodriguez-Chavez has been corrected as follows:

Current Affiliation Content:
Isaac R. Rodriguez-Chavez, PhD
Standards Association, Clinical
Trial Technology Modernization

The updated version of this book can be found at
https://doi.org/10.1007/978-3-031-62877-1

Network
CEO & Principal Independent
Consultant, 4Biosolutions Consulting Scientific, Clinical,
Regulatory Affairs and Digital
Health Technologies Editor,
Regulatory Science, DIA Global
Forum, Institute of Electrical and
Electronics
Rockville, MD, USA

Updated Affiliation Content:
Isaac R. Rodriguez-Chavez, PhD
CEO & Principal Independent Consultant, Scientific, Clinical, Regulatory Affairs and Digital Health Technologies, 4Biosolutions Consulting, Rockville, MD, USA

The affiliation for the author Craig Lipset has been corrected as follows:

Current Affiliation Content:
Craig Lipset
Decentralized Trials and Research Alliance
San Diego, CA, USA
Clinical Innovation, Pfizer
New York City, NY, USA

Updated Affiliation Content:
Craig Lipset
Decentralized Trials and Research Alliance
San Diego, CA, USA
Former Head, Clinical Innovation, Pfizer
New York City, NY, USA

Chapter 2: Technology Landscape and Requirements
Chapter 4: Methodology and Protocol Development
Chapter 5: Goals and Metrics of Success

The affiliation for the author Isaac R. Rodriguez-Chavez has been corrected as follows:

Correction to: Fundamentals of Decentralized Clinical Trials   C3

Current Affiliation Content:
Isaac R. Rodriguez-Chavez
4Biosolutions Consulting, Scientific, Clinical, Regulatory Affairs and Digital Health Technologies, IEEE-SA, Clinical Trial Technology Modernization Network (CTTMN), Rockville, MD, USA

Updated Affiliation Content:
Isaac R. Rodriguez-Chavez
CEO & Principal Independent Consultant, Scientific, Clinical, Regulatory Affairs and Digital Health Technologies, 4Biosolutions Consulting. Rockville, MD, USA

Chapter 3: Regulatory Landscape
The affiliation for the authors Anna H. Yang and Isaac R. Rodriguez-Chavez has been corrected as follows:

Current Affiliation Content:
Isaac R. Rodriguez-Chavez
Genentech, A Member of the Roche Group,
South San Francisco, CA, USA

Anna H. Yang
4Biosolutions Consulting, Scientific, Clinical, Regulatory Affairs and Digital Health Technologies, IEEE-SA, Clinical Trial Technology Modernization Network (CTTMN), Rockville, MD, USA

Updated Affiliation Content:
Isaac R. Rodriguez-Chavez
CEO & Principal Independent Consultant, Scientific, Clinical, Regulatory Affairs and Digital Health Technologies, 4Biosolutions Consulting. Rockville, MD, USA

Anna H. Yang
Genentech, A Member of the Roche Group,
South San Francisco, CA, USA

Notes

"Digital health technology" (DHT) is used in place of "wearable" in this book. DHT is the proper regulatory terminology.

"Trial participant" is used instead of "patient" to ensure alignment with proper regulatory terminology.

The term "brick and mortar trials" may be used interchangeably with "traditional trials".

Key distinction between telehealth and telemedicine: Telemedicine refers to using technology to deliver actual clinical care at a distance, while telehealth covers the full range of health-related services and information that can be provided remotely through technology. Telemedicine typically refers specifically to remote clinical services like diagnosis, treatment, and monitoring of patients. It involves clinicians using telecommunications technology to provide care to patients who are physically separated from them. Common examples are doctor video visits and remote monitoring of vital signs. Telehealth is a broader term that includes telemedicine as well as other health-related services that use technology to improve and facilitate care. Examples of telehealth beyond clinical services include health education, administrative meetings, training health professionals, etc. So, in short: telemedicine is a component of the broader category of telehealth. Telemedicine refers specifically to remote clinical care, while telehealth encompasses that plus many other technologies and methods to deliver health information and education.

© The Editor(s) (if applicable) and The Author(s), under exclusive license to Springer Nature Switzerland AG 2024
A. H. Yang, I. R. Rodriguez-Chavez (eds.), *Fundamentals of Decentralized Clinical Trials*,
https://doi.org/10.1007/978-3-031-62877-1

Variations Across the US and the Ex-US Markets

Different DCT modalities will have different allowance statuses across countries. For example, consenting electronically to a study, also known as eConsent, is accepted in the U.S. but not accepted in France. Here is a table below of modalities with varying degrees of allowances worldwide. Note that this list is current as of January 2022.

Each country has its own framework of risk tolerance for certain DCT approaches. Across the board, it is evident that IMP supply and eConsent have the most acceptance. Participant-generated data such as ePRO and DHTs can result in scattered acceptance. Home sampling is more accepted than participant-generated data but is still a risky approach in ex-US countries.

Index

A
Adverse events (AEs), 29, 68
Analytics platforms (APs), 20
Anti-Amyloid Treatment in Asymptomatic Alzheimer's Disease (A4) trial, 11
Application programming interfaces (APIs), 20
Artificial intelligence (AI), 8, 23, 24, 30

B
Best practices for clinical trials, 72
Biden-Harris Administration's strategy, 23
Biotechnology Innovation Organization (BIO), 8
Brick and mortar trials, 77

C
Center for Information and Study on Clinical Research Participation (CISCRP) Participant Insights and Perceptions Survey, 2
Centers for Medicaid and Medicare Services (CMS), 3
Clinical decision support software, 39
Clinical outcome assessments (COA), 36
Clinical research associate, 51
Clinical research coordinator or manager, 51
Clinical research team, 50–52
Clinical trial data warehouse (CTDWH), 20
Clinical trial management system (CTMS), 19, 27
Clinical trials transformation initiative (CTTI), 7–9
Cloud computing platforms (CCP), 20
Co-investigator (Co-I), 51
Consolidated Appropriations Act of 2022, 36
Container Technologies (CTs Dockers), 20
Contract research organizations (CROs), 6, 8
Cost-effectiveness, 25

COVID-19 pandemic, 3, 11, 29, 35, 46, 53
  decentralized clinical trial to, 2–5
  regulatory adjustments, 38–40

D

Data collection, 73
Data connectivity, 65
Data integration, 25
Data Management Plan (DMP), 56
Data Management System (DMS), 19, 20
Data Warehouses and Repositories (DWRs), 20
Decentralized clinical trial (DCT), 29, 30, 50, 64
  affect the team, 52, 53
  to COVID-19 pandemic, 2–5
  definition and value, 41, 42
  design, 42
  draft guidance and beyond, 41
  early metrics of success, 65, 66
  eNPV of, 64
  ethics committees, 57–60
  financial, structural and strategic investments, 6, 7
  flexible protocol for, 53
    data sources, 56, 57
    inclusion and exclusion criteria, 56
    trial design, 55, 56
    trial objectives and trial endpoints, 54, 55
  industry trends, 9–12
  investigational reviews boards, 57–60
  and key digital health technologies, 7–9
  key performance indicators, 66–72
  responsibilities of investigator, 44
Decentralized clinical trials for drugs, biological products, and devices, 39
Decentralized trials and research alliance (DTRA), 8, 65
Delegation log, 43
Digital communication, 29
Digital endpoints, 36
Digital health technologies (DHTs), 8, 36, 77
  measurements, 30
  for remote data acquisition in clinical investigations, 39
Digital health tools, 7
Digital navigator, 51
Direct-to-participant (DtP) shipment, 7, 28
Disruptive Innovations to Modernize Clinical Research (DPHARM), 41
Diverse DCT approaches, 5
Diversity Plans to Improve Enrollment of Participants from Underrepresented Racial and Ethnic Populations in Clinical Trials, 39

E

Eastern Cooperative Oncology Group (ECOG), 54
eConsent, 78
eDiary, 28
Efficacy-effectiveness gap, 73
eHealth, 8
Electronic data capture (EDC), 19
Electronic health information (EHI), 24
Electronic health records (EHRs), 6, 19, 22, 25, 30, 64
Electronic patient reported outcomes (ePRO), 19
Enhancing diversity of clinical trial populations, 3

Equity diversity, and inclusion (EDI), 36
Ethics committees (ECs), 57–60
Exclusion criteria, 56
Expected Net Present Value (eNPV), 64

F
Findable, Accessible, Interoperable and Reusable (FAIR) principles, 18
in clinical trial, 18, 20, 21
First Patient In (FPI), 68
Food and Drug Administration (FDA), 3
Food and Drug Omnibus Reform Act of 2022 (FDORA), 37
Fully DCT, 4, 8, 9, 41

G
Global regulators, 3
Good clinical practice (GCP), 45
Good distribution practice (GDP), 58
Good manufacturing practice (GMP), 58
Good trials, 72

H
Healthcare providers (HCPs), 7, 42, 73
Health data interoperability, 21–24
Health information technology, 9
Health information technology for economic and clinical health (HITECH) Act, 22
Health Insurance Portability and Accountability Act (HIPAA), 21, 69
Home health care, 7
Home health nurses, 52
Hybrid DCT, 4, 8, 9, 41, 45

I
Inclusion criteria, 56
Institutional Review Boards (IRBs), 8
Interactive clinical trial, 10
Interoperability, definition of, 23
Interventional clinical research, 7
Investigational medical products (IMPs), 7, 44
Investigational Reviews Boards (IRB), 57–60
Investigator of a clinical investigation, 50

K
Key performance indicators (KPIs), 65, 66
adverse events (AEs), 68
compliance, 71
cost, 70
database lock timelines, 71
diversity and inclusion, 69, 70
inclusion of participants in clinical trial due to DCT Facility, 72
likelihood to engage in DCT, 66
participant dropout percentage due to participant decision, 67
participant load per site, 71
speed through enrollment rate, 68

L
Laboratory Information Management System (LIMS), 19
Last Patient In (LPI), 68
Login identification (ID), 26

M
Machine learning (ML), 8, 30
Mapping the Participant Journey, 65

Medable Task Force, 58–60
Medicare beneficiaries, 4
Metadata catalogs (MCs), 20
Metadata repository (MDR), 20
Mobile Clinical Trials (MCT) Program, 9
Mobile health, 8
Modernizing Clinical Trial Conduct (MCTC), 52
Multi-Regional Clinical Trials (MRCT) Leadership Task Force, 58–60

N
Non-electronic case report forms (eCRF), 56
Non-interventional clinical research, 7
Nonmodifiable structural and clinical barriers, 2
Non-trial personnel, 43, 44

O
Observational study, 7
Ontology Management Systems (OMS), 20
Operational Complexity Assessment Tool (OCAT), 52

P
Participant-focused drug development, 3
Participant-reported outcomes (PROs), 67
Pharmaceutical Research and Manufacturers of America (PhRMA), 8
Pre COVID-19 pandemic, regulatory stage, 36, 37
Primary Investigator of a grant, 50
Protected health information (PHI), 21

R
Randomization and blinding system (RBS), 19
Randomized controlled trials (RCTs), 72
Regulatory landscape
 adjustments during COVID-19 pandemic, 38–40
 FDA DCT draft guidance and beyond, 41–44, 46
 pre COVID-19 pandemic, regulatory stage, 36, 37
Regulatory stage pre COVID-19 pandemic, 36, 37
REMOTE trial, 10
Research nurses, 51
Research pharmacists, 51

S
Safety reporting system (SRS), 19
Semantic Web Technologies (SWTs), 21
Serious adverse events (SAEs), 68
Service support, 52
Socioeconomic status (SES), 2
Sponsor-delegates, 29
Statistical analysis system (SAS), 19
Sub-investigator, 51

T
Task Log, 43
Technology implementation considerations, 25
 components, 26–29
Technology Modernization Action Plan (TMAP), 36
Telehealth, 7, 27, 43, 44, 77
Telemedicine, 36, 77
Trial participant, 77
Trial participant-reported information, 28

Trials@Home Initiative, 38
Trusted Exchange Framework and Common Agreement network (TEFCA), 24

U
Unique and persistent identifiers (UPIs), 20
US-based efforts to harmonize adoption, 21–24

V
Vendors, 73
Virtual research coordinator, 52

W
Web-based questionnaires, 10
Workflow management systems (WMS), 20
World Health Organization (WHO), 72

SPRINGER NATURE

GPSR Compliance

The European Union's (EU) General Product Safety Regulation (GPSR) is a set of rules that requires consumer products to be safe and our obligations to ensure this.

If you have any concerns about our products, you can contact us on ProductSafety@springernature.com

In case Publisher is established outside the EU, the EU authorized representative is:

Springer Nature Customer Service Center GmbH
Europaplatz 3
69115 Heidelberg, Germany

The manufacturer's authorised representative in the EU is Springer Nature Customer Service Centre GmbH, Europaplatz 3, 69115 Heidelberg, Germany. If you have any concerns regarding our products, please contact ProductSafety@springernature.com

Printed and bound by CPI Group (UK) Ltd, Croydon, CR0 4YY
25/03/2026
02078192-0001